Occupational Therapy Practice Guidelines for

Older Adults With Low Vision

Jennifer Kaldenberg, MSA, OTR/L, SCLV, FAOTA
Assistant Professor & Academic Fieldwork Coordinator
Boston University
Boston

Adjunct Assistant Professor of Vision Rehabilitation
New England College of Optometry
Boston

Stacy Smallfield, DrOT, OTR/L
Associate Professor
Department of Occupational Therapy
University of South Dakota
Vermillion

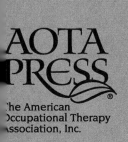
AOTA PRESS
The American
Occupational Therapy
Association, Inc.

AOTA Centennial Vision

We envision that occupational therapy is a powerful, widely recognized, science-driven, and evidence-based profession with a globally connected and diverse workforce meeting society's occupational needs.

AOTA Vision Statement

The American Occupational Therapy Association advances occupational therapy as the pre-eminent profession in promoting the health, productivity, and quality of life of individuals and society through the therapeutic application of occupation.

AOTA Mission Statement

The American Occupational Therapy Association advances the quality, availability, use, and support of occupational therapy through standard-setting, advocacy, education, and research on behalf of its members and the public.

AOTA Staff

Frederick P. Somers, *Executive Director*
Christopher M. Bluhm, *Chief Operating Officer*

Chris Davis, *Director, AOTA Press*
Ashley Hofmann, *Development/Production Editor*
Victoria Davis, *Digital/Production Editor*

Beth Ledford, *Director, Marketing*
Amanda Fogle, *Marketing Specialist*
Jennifer Folden, *Marketing Specialist*

The American Occupational Therapy Association, Inc.
4720 Montgomery Lane
Bethesda, MD 20814
301-652-AOTA (2682)
TDD: 800-377-8555
Fax: 301-652-7711
www.aota.org

To order: 1-877-404-AOTA (2682)

Disclaimers

This publication is designed to provide accurate and authoritative information in regard to the subject matter covered. It is sold or distributed with the understanding that the publisher is not engaged in rendering legal, accounting, or other professional service. If legal advice or other expert assistance is required, the services of a competent professional person should be sought.
—*From the Declaration of Principles jointly adopted by the American Bar Association and a Committee of Publishers and Associations*

It is the objective of the American Occupational Therapy Association to be a forum for free expression and interchange of ideas. The opinions expressed by the contributors to this work are their own and not necessarily those of the American Occupational Therapy Association.

ISBN-13: 978-1-56900-342-8
Library of Congress Control Number: 2013936591

Cover design by Jennifer Folden
Composition by Maryland Composition, Laurel, MD
Printing by Automated Graphics Systems, White Plains, MD

Contents

Best Practices and Summaries of Evidence

Appendixes

Figures, Tables, and Boxes Used in This Publication

Acknowledgments

The series editor for this Practice Guideline is

Deborah Lieberman, MHSA, OTR/L, FAOTA
Director, Evidence-Based Practice
Staff Liaison to the Commission on Practice
American Occupational Therapy Association
Bethesda, MD

The issue editor for this Practice Guideline is

Marian Arbesman, PhD, OTR/L
President, ArbesIdeas, Inc.
Consultant, AOTA Evidence-Based Practice Project
Clinical Assistant Professor, Department of
   Rehabilitation Science
State University of New York at Buffalo

The authors acknowledge the following individuals for their contributions to the evidence-based literature review:

Sue Berger, PhD, OTR/L, BCG, FAOTA
Melodie Brost, MS, OTR
Vanessa Horton, MS, OTR
Michael D. Justiss, PhD, OTR
Sarah Kenyon, MS, OTR
Chiung-ju Liu, PhD, OTR
Jessica McAteer, MS, OTR/L
Kristen Mears, MS, OTR
Ashley Myers, MS, OTR/L
Kari Clem, MS, OTR/L
Kara Schreier, MS, OTR/L

Jeff Butler, Chelsea Listenfelt, Nick Rush, and Julie Stover, who were graduate students at Indiana University at the time of this work.

The authors acknowledge and thank the following individuals for their participation in the content review and development of this publication:

Beth Barstow, PhD, OTR/L, SCLV
Sue Berger, PhD, OTR/L, BCG, FAOTA
Chiung-ju Liu, PhD, OTR
Julie Ann Nastasi, OTD, OTR/L, SCLV
Monica S. Perlmutter, OTD, OTR/L, SCLV
Jennifer Bogenrief, JD
V. Judith Thomas, MGA
Madalene Palmer

The authors thank the following individuals for their contribution:

Gina Bargioni, MS, OTR/L
Shannon Chovan, MS, OTR/L
Lizbeth Metzger, MS, OTR/L
Jill Palladino, MS, OTR/L

Note. The authors of this Practice Guideline have signed a Conflict of Interest statement indicating that they have no conflicts that would bear on this work.

Introduction

Purpose and Use of This Publication

Practice guidelines have been widely developed in response to the U.S. health care reform movement. Such guidelines can be a useful tool for improving the quality of health care, enhancing consumer satisfaction, promoting appropriate use of services, and reducing costs. The American Occupational Therapy Association (AOTA), which represents nearly 140,000 occupational therapists, occupational therapy assistants (see Appendix A), and students of occupational therapy, is committed to providing information to support decision making that promotes a high-quality health care system that is affordable and accessible to all.

Using an evidence-based perspective and key concepts from the second edition of the *Occupational Therapy Practice Framework: Domain and Process* (AOTA, 2008), this guideline provides an overview of the occupational therapy process for older adults with low vision. It defines the occupational therapy domain and process and interventions that occur within the boundaries of acceptable practice. This guideline does not discuss all possible methods of care, and although it does recommend some specific methods of care, the occupational therapist makes the ultimate judgment regarding the appropriateness of a given intervention in light of a specific person's circumstances and needs and the evidence available to support the intervention.

It is the intention of AOTA, through this publication, to help occupational therapists and occupational therapy assistants, as well as those people who manage, reimburse, or set policy regarding occupational therapy services, understand the contribution of occupational therapy in treating older adults with low vision. This guideline also can serve as a reference for health care professionals, health care facility managers, education and health care regulators, third-party payers, and managed care organizations. Selected diagnostic and billing code information for evaluations and interventions is provided in Appendix B.

This document may be used in any of the following ways:

- To assist occupational therapists and occupational therapy assistants in communicating about their services to external audiences
- To assist eye care professionals, other health care practitioners, case managers, families and caregivers, and health care facility managers in determining whether referral for occupational therapy services would be appropriate
- To assist third-party payers in determining the medical necessity for occupational therapy
- To assist legislators, third-party payers, and administrators in understanding the professional education, training, and skills of occupational therapists and occupational therapy assistants
- To assist health and education planning teams in determining the need for occupational therapy
- To assist program developers, administrators, legislators, and third-party payers in understanding the scope of occupational therapy services
- To assist program evaluators and policy analysts in this practice area in determining outcome measures for analyzing the effectiveness of occupational therapy intervention
- To assist policy, education, and health care benefit analysts in understanding the

appropriateness of occupational therapy services for older adults with low vision

- To assist policymakers, legislators, and organizations in understanding the contribution occupational therapy can make in program development and health care reform for older adults with low vision
- To assist occupational therapy educators in designing appropriate curricula that incorporate the role of occupational therapy with older adults with low vision.

The introduction to this guideline continues with a brief discussion of the domain and process of occupational therapy. This discussion is followed by a detailed description of the occupational therapy process for older adults with low vision, including a summary of evidence from the literature regarding best practices with this population. Embedded in these descriptions are summaries of the results of systematic reviews of evidence from the scientific literature regarding best practices in occupational therapy intervention for older adults with low vision. Finally, the appendixes contain the methodology (Appendix C) and evidence tables (Appendix D) for the review and guidelines related to using *Current Procedural Terminology™ (CPT)* codes for billing (Appendix B).

Domain and Process of Occupational Therapy

Occupational therapy practitioners' expertise lies in their knowledge of occupation and of how engaging in occupations can be used to support health and participation in home, school, the workplace, and community life (AOTA, 2008).

In 2008, the AOTA Representative Assembly adopted the *Occupational Therapy Practice Framework: Domain and Process* (2nd ed.). Informed by the first edition of the *Occupational Therapy Practice Framework:* (AOTA, 2002), the previous *Uniform Terminology for Occupational Therapy* (AOTA, 1979, 1989, 1994), and the World Health Organization's (WHO's) *International Classification of Functioning, Disability and Health (ICF;* WHO, 2001), the *Framework* outlines the profession's domain and the process of service delivery within this domain.

Domain

A profession's *domain* articulates its sphere of knowledge, societal contribution, and intellectual or scientific activity. The occupational therapy profession's domain centers on helping others participate in daily life activities. The broad term that the profession uses to describe daily life activities is *occupation.* As outlined in the *Framework,* occupational therapists and occupational therapy assistants[1] work collaboratively with people, organizations, and populations (clients) to engage in everyday activities or occupations that they want and need to do in a manner that supports health and participation (see Figure 1). Using occupational engagement as both the desired outcome of intervention and the intervention itself, occupational therapy practitioners[2] are skilled at viewing the subjective and objective aspects of performance and understanding occupation simultaneously from this dual, yet holistic, perspective. The overarching mission to support health and participation in life through engagement in occupations circumscribes the profession's domain and emphasizes the important ways in which environmental and life circumstances influence the manner in which people carry out their occupations. Key

---

[1]*Occupational therapists* are responsible for all aspects of occupational therapy service delivery and are accountable for the safety and effectiveness of the occupational therapy service delivery process. *Occupational therapy assistants* deliver occupational therapy services under the supervision of and in partnership with an occupational therapist (AOTA, 2009).

[2]When the term *occupational therapy practitioner* is used in this document, it refers to both occupational therapists and occupational therapy assistants (AOTA, 2006).

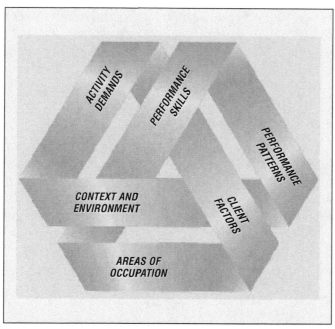

Figure 1. Occupational therapy's domain.

Reprinted from "Occupational Therapy Practice Framework: Domain and Process" (2nd ed., p. 627), by American Occupational Therapy Association, 2008, *American Journal of Occupational Therapy, 62,* 625–683. Used with permission.

aspects of the domain of occupational therapy are defined in Figure 2.

Process

Many professions use the process of evaluating, intervening, and targeting outcomes that is outlined in the *Framework.* Occupational therapy's application of this process is made unique, however, by its focus on occupation (see Figure 3). The process of occupational therapy service delivery typically begins with the *occupational profile*—an assessment of the client's occupational needs, problems, and concerns—and the *analysis of occupational performance,* which includes the skills, patterns, contexts and environments, activity demands, and client factors that contribute to or impede the client's satisfaction with his or her ability to engage in valued daily life activities. Therapists then plan and implement intervention using a variety of approaches and methods in which occupation is both the means and the ends (Trombly, 1995).

Occupational therapists continually assess the effectiveness of the intervention and the client's progress toward targeted outcomes. The intervention review informs decisions to continue or discontinue intervention and to make referrals to other agencies or professionals.

AREAS OF OCCUPATION	CLIENT FACTORS	PERFORMANCE SKILLS	PERFORMANCE PATTERNS	CONTEXT AND ENVIRONMENT	ACTIVITY DEMANDS
Activities of Daily Living (ADL)* Instrumental Activities of Daily Living (IADL) Rest and Sleep Education Work Play Leisure Social Participation *Also referred to as *basic activities of daily living (BADL)* or *personal activities of daily living (PADL).*	Values, Beliefs, and Spirituality Body Functions Body Structures	Sensory Perceptual Skills Motor and Praxis Skills Emotional Regulation Skills Cognitive Skills Communication and Social Skills	Habits Routines Roles Rituals	Cultural Personal Physical Social Temporal Virtual	Objects Used and Their Properties Space Demands Social Demands Sequencing and Timing Required Actions Required Body Functions Required Body Structures

Figure 2. Aspects of occupational therapy's domain.

Reprinted from "Occupational Therapy Practice Framework: Domain and Process" (2nd ed., p. 628), by American Occupational Therapy Association, 2008, *American Journal of Occupational Therapy, 62,* 625–683. Used with permission.

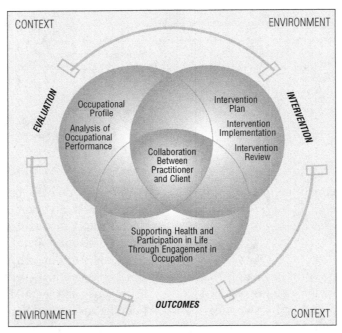

Figure 3. Occupational therapy's process of service delivery as applied within the profession's domain.

Reprinted from "Occupational Therapy Practice Framework: Domain and Process" (2nd ed., p. 627), by American Occupational Therapy Association, (2008), *American Journal of Occupational Therapy, 62,* 625–683. Used with permission.

Overview of Occupational Therapy for Adults With Low Vision

Definition and Epidemiology

The U.S. population is aging, and occupational therapy practitioners working with older adults must have the skills to address multiple health issues, one of which is vision loss. Although typical aging does not cause low vision, four major causes of visual impairment are directly related to the aging process: (1) age-related macular degeneration (AMD), (2) diabetic retinopathy, (3) glaucoma, and (4) cataracts.

The number of adults diagnosed with AMD is expected to double to 17.8 million by 2050 (Rein et al., 2009), and the number of adults diagnosed with diabetic retinopathy is expected to increase to 9.9 million in that same time frame (Saaddine et al., 2008). The number of people with glaucoma in the United States is 2.2 million and is expected to increase to 3 million by 2020 (National Eye Institute [NEI], 2011). Additionally, more than 30 million adults are expected to be diagnosed with cataracts by 2020 (Congdon et al., 2004). Of the clients seen for low vision rehabilitation services, nearly 1 in 3 is ages 80 or older (Owsley, McGwin, Lee, Wasserman, & Searcey, 2009). Clearly, visual impairment in the older adult population is a significant public health issue that requires attention.

Although no commonly accepted standard definition of low vision exists (Owsley et al., 2009), the term is used to describe the vast gray area between normal vision and total blindness (Stuen & Faye, 2003). *Low vision* is typically defined as visual acuity worse than 20/60 when using best correction, a visual field loss, or both (Centers for Medicare and Medicaid Services [CMS], 2002). Low vision is not caused by a single condition but rather by any of a number of disease processes that produce decreased visual acuity or visual field bilaterally. Additionally, these visual impairments cannot be corrected through the use of medication, corrective lenses, or surgery (NEI, n.d.).

For medical insurance reimbursement purposes, low vision is limited to visual impairments that meet the *International Classification of Diseases* (9th rev., clinicial modification; [*ICD–9–CM*]; *World Health Organization,* 1999) diagnostic criteria for reduced visual acuity, visual field, or both (CMS, 2002). For further information regarding *ICD–9–CM* diagnostic criteria, refer to Table 1.

Legal blindness, however, is a severe level of visual impairment, defined as best corrected visual acuity of 20/200 in the better-seeing eye or a visual field of 20° or less (List of Impairments, 2006). The governmental description of the degree of visual impairment that qualifies one for government assistance and programs is based on the degree of visual loss, hence the term *legally blind.* It is important to note, though, that many older adults who are either legally blind or have low vision have residual, usable vision (Stuen & Faye, 2003).

Both low vision and legal blindness result in a person's decreased ability to carry out normal, everyday activities without adaptation or compensatory strategies. For example, tasks such as reading information on personal computers, telecommunication devices, medication prescriptions, financial statements, product labels, signage, recipes, and menus may be limited by low vision or legal blindness. Even at a mild visual impairment level in the range of 20/40 to 20/70, older adults may experience a significant decline in participation in everyday activities (Perlmutter, Bhorade, Gordon, Hollingsworth, & Baum, 2010). In other words, visual impairment can have a considerable impact on a person's ability to perform occupations of choice.

This Practice Guideline includes occupational therapy assessment and intervention guidelines for older adults who have visual acuity impairments, visual field impairments, or both as the result of a low vision diagnosis. Readers are referred to the *Occupational Therapy Practice Guidelines for Adults With Traumatic Brain Injury* (Golisz, 2009) and the *Occupational Therapy Practice Guidelines for Adults With Stroke* (Sabari, 2008) for assessment and intervention strategies when working with adults with a neurological visual impairment with resulting visual perception deficits.

The Aging Eye

Changes to the eye occur naturally, with normative aging beginning at about age 40. Typical aging changes include a thickening and yellowing of the lens and smaller pupil that result in the need for increased illumination (as much as 3–4 times greater illumination than a younger person) for vision-related activities (Figueiro, 2001; Stuen & Faye, 2003). Other changes include (1) loss of accommodation (commonly referred to as *presbyopia*), which often necessitates reading glasses; (2) a slight decline in visual acuity; (3) difficulty with glare; (4) slower adaptation to light and dark; (5) reduced contrast sensitivity; and (6) reduced depth perception, all of which make nighttime seeing, and driving, more difficult (Figueiro, 2001; Stuen & Faye, 2003).

Age-Related Eye Diseases

Unlike normative age-related changes in the eye, visual acuity that cannot be corrected to 20/60 or better, blind or blurry spots in the central vision (central scotomas), a constricted visual field, or bilateral field cuts are not typical (Stuen & Faye, 2003). Rather, these changes may be indications of uncorrectable vision impairments that fall into the category of low vision. Age-related eye diseases can be divided into categories on the basis of the type of impairments they cause
- Central visual field impairment
- Peripheral field impairment
- Mixed visual field loss.

Central Visual Field Impairment

The central 20° of the visual field (the macula) is where the best visual acuity is located. Therefore, a loss of central vision implies a decreased ability to see clearly (Weisser-Pike & Kaldenberg, 2010). It is the most common deficit seen in low vision rehabilitation services (Owsley et al., 2009). Age-related eye diseases that cause central field visual impairment include AMD and cataracts, and older adults with these diagnoses describe their vision as blurry, fuzzy, or cloudy because they develop a *scotoma*, or blind spot, in their central visual field. Functionally, this scotoma leads to a decreased ability to see fine detail, read, drive, recognize faces, and detect colors accurately.

Age-Related Macular Degeneration

AMD is a progressive and irreversible loss of central vision caused by a breakdown or atrophy of the photoreceptors located in the macula (NEI, 2009a). It is the most common cause of visual impairment in the United States (Owsley et al., 2009). There are two types of AMD: wet and dry. The dry form, also called *nonexudative AMD,* is the more common form, accounting for more than 85% of moderate to severe AMD cases (NEI, 2009a). The wet form, or *exudative AMD*, is an advanced type of AMD caused by the abnormal development of blood vessels that leak fluid. Common medical interventions for wet AMD include anti–vascular endothelial growth factor treatments, photodynamic therapy, and laser surgery, which are typically limited to those with wet AMD; therefore, only a very small percentage of those with the disease benefit from medical intervention (NEI, 2009a).

A variety of medical and nutritional interventions are used to treat AMD; however, they are not discussed here because they are outside the scope of this Practice Guideline. The majority of individuals with AMD have a permanent decrease in visual acuity and visual field that limits the ability to perform meaningful daily activities effectively and efficiently.

Cataract

A *cataract* is an opacity of the crystalline lens (NEI, 2009b). If one lives long enough, one will develop cataracts; however, cataracts are treatable through surgery. When a cataract forms, it causes light rays that enter the eye to scatter, causing glare and discomfort. Other symptoms include decreased visual acuity, decreased contrast sensitivity, difficulty with nighttime driving, and complaints of diplopia or double vision. A cataract is generally considered for removal when it begins to interfere with occupational performance, at which time the human crystalline lens is removed and replaced with a new intraocular lens (NEI, 2009b). However, some individuals may not be surgical candidates, and in that case the cataract can have an impact on all aspects of function.

Peripheral Visual Field Impairment

The peripheral visual system is what people use to gather information about their broader spatial environment. It detects large objects and movement within the environment that then signal one's attention. Unlike central vision, the peripheral vision has a lower visual acuity. A loss of peripheral vision causes *tunnel vision*, or a constricted field of view. Eye diseases that cause peripheral field visual impairment include glaucoma and hemianopsia or quadrantanopsia as the result of stroke or traumatic brain injury. Functionally, this impairment causes difficulties with navigation (bumping into objects or people) during both day and night and with reaching for commonly used objects.

Glaucoma

Glaucoma is a group of diseases that cause abnormal fluid pressure on the optic nerve, which causes loss of peripheral vision (NEI, n.d.). Damage can occur through increased pressure resulting from poor drainage through the anterior chamber of the eye or closure of the angle (NEI, n.d.). People at increased risk of developing glaucoma are African Americans, people older than age 60, and people with a family history of glaucoma (NEI, n.d.).

Primary *open-angle glaucoma* can be treated with medications, surgical intervention, or a combination; *closed-angle glaucoma* needs immediate medical intervention or it can lead to complete blindness (NEI, n.d.). Medications used to treat glaucoma need to be taken as prescribed, and patients need to understand that even though they may be asymptomatic, following their prescribed medication regime is important.

Hemianopsia and Quadrantanopsia

Visual field impairments often associated with stroke or traumatic brain injury include hemianopsia or quadrantanopsia. Vision impairment is reported to occur in 36% of people with right-hemisphere stroke and 25% of people with left-hemisphere stroke (Wolter & Preda, 2006). In addition, the visual field impairment (nasal, temporal, superior, inferior) is specific to the area of the brain that is involved. Optometrists or ophthalmologists may use prisms or visual training to improve awareness of the visual field (Bowers, Keeney, & Peli, 2008). For more information on the occupational therapy practitioner's role in addressing neurological visual field impairment, we refer readers to the *Occupational Therapy Practice Guidelines for Adults With Traumatic Brain Injury* (Golisz, 2009) and the *Occupational Therapy Practice Guidelines for Adults With Stroke* (Sabari, 2008).

Mixed Visual Field Loss

Mixed visual field loss occurs when both the central and the peripheral visual fields are affected by disease or injury. Many diseases may be associated with mixed visual field loss; however, the most common conditions that occupational therapy practitioners encounter include diabetic retinopathy, multiple sclerosis, and hypertension. Mixed visual field loss functionally affects the ability to see fine detail and the ability to detect changes in the environment. Therefore, its impact on daily function can be quite severe. In addition, a person with mixed visual field loss may experience variable visual impairment, which is dependent on physiological or environmental conditions. For example, variable lighting conditions may have a significant effect on function for a person with mixed visual field loss.

Diabetic Retinopathy

Diabetic retinopathy is a common example of mixed visual field loss. Diabetic retinopathy affects 40%–45% of all individuals with diabetes (NEI, 2009c). There are two types of diabetic retinopathy: (1) nonproliferative and (2) proliferative.

Diabetes affects the blood vessels in the retina. In *nonproliferative diabetic retinopathy*, the blood vessels in the retina swell or become occluded, which limits the blood supply to the retina, whereas in *proliferative diabetic retinopathy*, the occluded small blood vessels of the retina trigger the growth of new, abnormal blood vessels (NEI, 2009c). These new vessels often leak blood and other fluid, causing blurred vision or scotomas scattered throughout the visual field (NEI, 2009c). If left untreated, it can result in blindness (NEI, 2009c). Medical treatment for diabetic retinopathy includes surgery, laser treatments, and vitrectomy.

Occupational Therapy Process for Older Adults With Low Vision

Screening

Because of the prevalence of visual impairment in people older than age 65, regular screening of functional vision should be included in occupational therapy practice. The purpose of screening for functional vision is to identify visual deficits that may affect occupational performance and to initiate referral to the eye care practitioner. This screening typically is not reimbursed by third-party payers, yet it can identify a person in need of services and begin the referral process. Occupational therapists should screen the areas of visual function that have been found to increase a person's risk of functional impairment in addition to their standard assessment of other components of function. These areas include distance and near visual acuity, contrast sensitivity, and central and peripheral visual field (Ramrattan et al., 2001; Rubin, Roche, Prasada-Rao, & Fried, 1994; Taylor, 2002; Waern et al., 2002; Wang, Mitchell, Simpson, Cumming, & Smith, 2001; West et al., 2002).

One formal screening tool to identify whether an older adult may be in need of a low vision eye exam or rehabilitation services is the Functional Vision Screening Questionnaire (Horowitz, Teresi, & Cassels, 1991; Lighthouse International, 1996), a 15-item self-report tool that includes items regarding basic functional tasks such as reading the newspaper, mail, and medication labels that may be affected when experiencing vision loss. The individual simply answers "yes" or "no" to each of the 15 items. Each "yes" or "no" response has a corresponding score of either 0 or 1, depending on the question. The responses are totaled to give a total score on the screening tool, with scores ranging from 0 to 15. A person scoring 9 or more should be encouraged to seek professional assistance (Horowitz et al., 1991; Lighthouse International, 1996).

Referral

Before an occupational therapy low vision evaluation is initiated, it is important that an ophthalmologist, optometrist, or both address the client's ocular health. Occupational therapy assessment and intervention will be more accurate and effective if the client has his or her best corrected vision. For best practice, the client should have had a recent ocular health exam and comprehensive low vision assessment to maximize visual acuity and visual field through the use of prescription lenses or other medical intervention. Therefore, a referral to an appropriate eye care professional should be made before initiating therapy services to ensure that the client is prepared for occupational therapy assessment and intervention.

A referral for occupational therapy services for older adults with low vision is appropriate when the visual impairment begins to affect their engagement in occupations. A referral may be generated by an eye care professional, a physician, another health care practitioner, a family member, or the client himself or herself. Occupational therapy's unique focus on engagement in valued occupations and roles to promote participation in one's home and community is an integral component of multidisciplinary rehabilitative services provided in a variety of facility- and community-based treatment programs. Older adults with low vision who reside in the community in independent or supportive environments may request referral to intermittent occupational therapy services for a variety of reasons over the course of the disease process.

When a referral is received, the occupational therapist must ensure that it is medically necessary and appropriate so that third-party payers will reimburse for the occupational therapy services provided. The CMS, a common third-party payer for occupational therapy services in low vision rehabilitation, has outlined the level of impairment needed in the better eye and the lesser eye to qualify for low vision rehabilitation services (CMS, 2002;

Colenbrander & Fletcher, 1995). Level of impairment ranges from *total blindness*, defined as no light perception, to *moderate visual impairment*, which is a best corrected visual acuity of less than 20/60. At a minimum, both the better eye and the lesser eye must have at least moderate visual impairment to qualify for Medicare reimbursement of occupational therapy services for low vision (CMS, 2002). Additionally, a bilateral field deficit, either homonymous or heteronymous; generalized constriction; or a central scotoma also qualify a person for skilled therapeutic services that are reimbursable by CMS (CMS, 2002). Table 1 lists the common *ICD-9*

Table 1. *ICD-9-CM* Diagnostic Codes Specific to Low Vision Rehabilitation

Lesser Eye	Better Eye				
	Total Impairment, No Light Perception	Near Total Impairment, >20/1,000 or <5°	Profound Impairment, 20/500–20/1,000 or <10°	Severe Impairment, <20/160–20/400 or <20°	Moderate Impairment, <20/60–20/160
1. Total impairment, no light perception	369.01	369.03	369.06	369.12	369.16
2. Near total impairment, >20/1,000 or <5°		369.04	369.07	369.13	369.17
3. Profound impairment, 20/500–20/1,000 or <10°			369.08	369.14	369.18
4. Severe impairment, <20/160–20/400 or <20°				369.22	369.24
5. Moderate impairment, <20/60–20/160					369.25
Central scotoma					368.41
Generalized contraction or constriction					368.45
Homonymous bilateral field defect					368.46
Heteronymous bilateral field defect					368.47

Note. How to use this chart: First, locate the visual impairment level of the better eye in the column headings. Then, to locate the correct *ICD-9* code, follow that column down to the row that contains the visual impairment level of the worse eye. *Example:* better eye = 20/200 and worse eye = 20/1000. Locate the severe impairment column along the top; follow it down to the profound impairment row. The correct *ICD-9* code would be 369.14. *ICD-9 = International Classification of Diseases* (9th rev.).
Source. This chart is adapted from Colenbrander (2002) and the *ICD-9-Clinical Modification* (WHO, 1999).

---

diagnostic codes specific to low vision rehabilitation on the basis of the level of visual impairment in both the better and the lesser eye. Box 1 provides an example of an older adult, Lillian, who was referred to occupational therapy services for low vision rehabilitation and discusses whether she qualifies for services on the basis of her level of visual impairment.

Evaluation

Occupational therapists perform evaluations in collaboration with the client and target information specific to the desired outcomes. The two elements of the occupational therapy evaluation are (1) the occupational profile and (2) the analysis of occupational performance (AOTA, 2008). Occupational therapists working with older adults with low vision may use standardized and nonstandardized assessments that are specifically designed for use with this population. Occupational therapists should validate clinical observations with data from standardized assessments. Consistent use of standardized assessments across the continuum of care during the disease process enhances continuity of care and allows for retrospective analysis of client outcomes, contributing to the evidence supporting practice. Table 2 provides a brief overview of selected assessments that may be used with older adults with low vision.

Occupational Profile

The purpose of the occupational profile is to determine who the client or clients are, identify their needs or concerns and to ascertain how these concerns affect engagement in occupational performance. Information for the occupational profile is gathered through formal and informal interviews with the client and significant others. Formal

Table 2. Selected Assessments Used by Occupational Therapists in Low Vision Rehabilitation

Specific Functions Within Aspects of the Domain of Occupational Therapy	Examples of Specific Assessments Used in Low Vision Rehabilitation
Areas of occupation	
• Activities of daily living • Instrumental activities of daily living • Rest and sleep • Education • Work • Leisure • Social participation	• Canadian Occupational Performance Measure (COPM; Law et al., 2005) • Activity Card Sort (ACS; Baum & Edwards, 2008) • Functional Vision Screening Questionnaire (Horowitz, Teresi, & Cassels, 1991) • Impact of Vision Impairment (Lamoureax, Hassell, & Keeffe, 2004) • Melbourne Low-Vision ADL Index (Haymes, Johnston, & Heyes, 2001) • Structured observation of activity • Driver performance testing • Role checklist • Leisure interest checklist
Performance skills	
• Communication and social skills	• MNRead Acuity Charts (Mansfield, Legge, Luebker, & Cunningham, 1994) • Pepper Visual Skills for Reading Test (Watson, Whittaker, & Steciw, 1995) • Morgan Low Vision Reading Comprehension Assessment (Watson, Wright, & Long, 1996) • Low Vision Writing Assessment (Watson, Wright, Wyse, & De l'Aune, 2004) • Brain Injury Visual Assessment Battery for Adults (biVABA; Warren, 1998)
• Motor and praxis skills	• Berg Balance Scale (Berg, Wood-Dauphinee, & Williams, 1995) • Functional Reach (Duncan, Weiner, Chandler, & Studenski, 1990) • Timed Up and Go (Podsiadlo & Richardson, 1991) • Tinetti Performance Oriented Mobility Assessment (Tinetti, 1986)
• Emotional regulation skills	• Center for Epidemiologic Studies Depression Scale (Radloff, 1977) • Geriatric Depression Scale (Yesavage et al., 1982–1983)
• Cognitive skills	• Mini-Mental State Examination (Folstein, Folstein, & McHugh, 1975) • Short Blessed Test (Katzman et al., 1983) • Montreal Cognitive Assessment (Nasreddine, 2011) • Loewenstein Occupational Therapy Cognitive Assessment (Itzkovish, Elazar, & Averbuch, 1990) • Cognitive Assessment of Minnesota (Rustad et al., 1993)
• Sensory–perceptual skills	• Standardized sensory testing (Bentzel, 2008)
Performance patterns	
• Habits, routines, and rituals and roles	• ACS (Baum & Edwards, 2008) • Interview • Observation of areas of occupation
Contexts and environments	
• Personal, physical, social, cultural, temporal, and virtual context and environments in which client is expected to perform activities and roles	• COPM (Law et al., 2005) • Home Environment Lighting Assessment (Perlmutter, n.d.) • Structured home safety assessment
Activity demands	
• Physical, spatial, social, and temporal requirements of activities client wants to or is expected to perform	• Observational assessment during task performance • Interview

(Continued)

Table 2. Selected Assessments Used by Occupational Therapists in Low Vision Rehabilitation *(Cont.)*

Specific Functions Within Aspects of the Domain of Occupational Therapy	Examples of Specific Assessments Used in Low Vision Rehabilitation
Client factors	
• Visual acuity	• Near acuity
	• Distance acuity
	• Many commercially available, both near and distance acuity test charts included in biVABA (Warren, 1998)
• Contrast sensitivity	• Contrast Sensitivity Chart (biVABA; Warren, 1998)
	• Peripheral visual field
	• Central visual field
	• Confrontation testing (Scheiman, 2002; biVABA [Warren, 1998])
	• Cancellation tests
• Visual field	• Observation (biVABA; Warren, 1998)
• Oculomotor Control Fixation	
• Tracking (Quintana, 2008; Scheiman, 2002)	
• Smooth pursuits (Garzia, Richman, Nicholson, & Gaines, 1990; Kulp & Schmidt, 1997; Maples, Atchley, & Ficklin, 1992; Scheiman, 2002)	
• Ocular motility (Maples et al., 1992; Quintana, 2008; Scheiman, 2002)	
• Binocular Vision Eye Alignment (Quintana, 2008)	• Observation biVABA (Warren, 1998)
• Convergence Accommodation (Quintana, 2008; Scheiman, 2002)	
• Smooth pursuits (Garzia et al., 1990; Kulp & Schmidt, 1997; Maples et al., 1992; Scheiman, 2002)	
• Saccades (Garzia et al., 1990; Kulp & Schmidt, 1997; Maples et al., 1992; Scheiman, 2002)	

assessments may include the Canadian Occupational Performance Measure (COPM; Law & Baum, 1998) or the Activity Card Sort (Baum & Edwards, 2008).

Conversations with the client help the occupational therapist gain perspective on how the client spends his or her time; what activities the client wants or needs to do; and how the environment in which the client lives, works, and participates in leisure and social activities supports or hinders occupational engagement. Developing the occupational profile involves the following steps:

- Identify the client or clients.
- Determine why the client is seeking services. Through interviews or checklists, the occupational therapist assists the client in identifying the current concerns relative to the areas of occupation and performance. The client's ability to identify and establish goals is essential to the rehabilitative process. Clients with decreased awareness of or insight into the permanence of the visual impairment may not be aware of its impact on their occupational performance.
- Identify the areas of occupation that are successful and the areas that are causing problems or risks. On the basis of the client's current concerns, the occupational therapist identifies possible visual impairments (e.g., visual acuity, visual field, contrast sensitivity) and environmental barriers and current supports related to occupational performance.
- Discuss significant aspects of the client's occupational history. Significant aspects can include

Lillian struggles with adjusting to her visual changes but has great social and emotional supports. Lillian was an avid reader and would like to be able to return to reading for home management skills and leisure. She is able to manage her activities of daily living tasks but struggles with instrumental activities of daily living tasks that require reading: financial management and medication management.

Lillian lives alone in a single-family home, with multiple floors, in an urban area and has family who live nearby.

Lillian's goals:
- Independence in money management
- Independence in medication management
- Independence in meal preparation and cooking for herself and her family
- Independence in reading for leisure.

life experiences (e.g., medical interventions, employment history, vocational preferences), occupational roles, interests, and previous patterns of engagement in occupations that provide meaning to the client's life.
- Determine the client's priorities and desired outcomes. Throughout the rehabilitative process, the occupational therapist and the client will discuss and prioritize goals so that the therapist's evaluation and interventions will match the client's desired outcomes. At times, the occupational therapist may need to refer the client to additional professionals or resources to achieve successful outcomes.

Box 2 provides an example of an occupational profile for an older adult, Lillian, with low vision.

Analysis of Occupational Performance

The occupational therapist uses information from the occupational profile to focus on the specific areas of occupation and the context and environment in which the client will live and function.

When the occupational therapist is able to analyze occupational performance, the following steps are generally included:
- Observe the client as he or she performs the occupations in the natural or least restrictive

environment (when possible), and note the effectiveness of the client's performance skills (e.g., sensory–perceptual, cognitive, emotional regulation, communication, social) and performance patterns (e.g., habits, routines, rituals, roles).
- Select specific assessments and evaluation methods that will identify and measure the factors related to the specific aspects of the domain of practice that may be influencing the client's performance. These assessments may focus on the client's body structures and functions, activity performance, or community participation. See Table 2 for examples of selected assessments.
- Interpret the assessment data to identify what supports or hinders performance.
- Develop or refine a hypothesis regarding the client's performance (i.e., identify underlying impairments or performance skill limitations that may be influencing occupational performance in multiple areas, such as visual field impairments affecting morning hygiene, home management tasks, community mobility, and social interaction).
- Develop goals in collaboration with the client and family, when relevant, that address the client's desired outcomes.

- Identify potential intervention approaches, guided by best practice and the evidence, and discuss them with the client, the client's family, or both.
- Document the evaluation process, and communicate the results to the appropriate team members and community agencies.

Areas of Occupation

Occupational therapists may elect to use an evaluation approach that focuses on possible impairments affecting performance of functional tasks (labeled a *bottom-up evaluation* by some occupational therapists) or an evaluation approach that begins by analyzing the roles of the individual with visual impairment and the areas of occupation that encompass the client's typical day (labeled a *top-down evaluation* by some occupational therapists). In the top-down evaluation approach, the occupational therapist performs a deeper analysis of underlying impairments contributing to activity limitations and participation restrictions only if he or she observes difficulty during performance of the actual occupation. Using a bottom-up approach, the occupational therapist focuses on the client's impairments and generic abilities and makes inferences as to how they might affect performance in present and future occupations.

The choice of evaluation approach is partially influenced by the client's ability to engage actively in the evaluation process. During the evaluation process, the occupational therapist may move between a top-down and a bottom-up approach, depending on the phase of recovery and the client's expressed desired outcomes.

Although standardized assessments exist that address activities of daily living (ADLs) and instrumental activities of daily living (IADLs), few address the unique needs of people with visual impairment. For example, the challenges associated with dressing tasks often involve the ability to locate, identify, and match articles of clothing rather than the ability to physically don and doff articles of clothing. Medication management may be difficult as a result of decreased ability to read medication labels or identify medications. For an older adult with diabetes, reading a blood glucose monitor or the markings on an insulin syringe may limit the ability to safely and independently perform this task. Bathing may be problematic because of the difficulty in distinguishing needed items in the bathroom or identifying the appropriate temperature setting on the dial. This kind of information cannot always be gleaned from typical occupational therapy ADL assessments such as the Functional Independence Measure (FIM™; Uniform Data System for Medical Rehabilitation, 1997) or the Barthel Index (Mahoney & Barthel, 1965).

Although several assessments may evaluate areas of occupation, three assessments specifically address the impact of vision loss on everyday activities and are discussed here (Haymes et al., 2001; Keefe, Lam, Cheung, Dinh, & McCarty, 1998; Lamoureux, Hassell, & Keefe, 2004). The Melbourne Low-Vision ADL Index (MLVAI) contains 27 items (of an original 74 items), broken into two categories: (1) self-care ADLs (9 items) and (2) IADLs (18 items; Haymes et al., 2001). The IADL items are measured by observing the client's performance of each task, whereas the self-care ADL items are assessed using a self-report format (Haymes et al., 2001). We should note that the MLVAI was developed in Australia, in an Australian context; therefore, the test kit is not readily available in the United States.

The Impact of Vision Impairment (IVI) assessment has 32 items that can be either self-administered or interviewer-administered (Lamoureux et al., 2004). The Self-Report Assessment of Functional Visual Performance Profile has an optional observation assessment of selected ADL and IADL tasks. The 38 tasks are rated on a 3-point scale: *unable, difficult,* or *independent* (Gilbert & Baker, 2011). Again, both of these instruments have undergone reliability and validity testing that demonstrated the appropriateness of their use in clinical settings (Gilbert & Baker, 2011; Haymes et al., 2001; Lamoureux et al., 2004).

When comparing these assessments, it is important to note that the MLVAI and the Self-Report Assessment of Functional Visual Performance Profile contain items that require actual performance of the task rather than relying on self-report alone (Gilbert & Baker, 2011; Haymes et al., 2001).

In addition, the COPM also has been cited as a useful outcome measure for clients with visual impairment (Pizzimenti & Roberts, 2005). The COPM is a semistructured interview in which the client identifies the top activities that he or she is having difficulty performing (Law et al., 1990; Law & Baum, 1998). The top five activities are then rated on a scale ranging from 1 to 10 on performance and satisfaction with performance. The Performance and Satisfaction subscales are each averaged for one score on a scale ranging from 1 to 10. "The COPM is designed to help occupational therapists clearly establish occupational performance goals based on client perceptions of need and to measure change objectively in defined problem areas" (Law et al., 1990, p. 84). It is a reliable and valid measure of occupational performance (McColl et al., 2006).

Please refer to Box 3 for an analysis of occupational performance as illustrated in the case study of Lillian.

Performance Skills

The evaluation of older adults with low vision includes assessing overt and subtle factors that may affect performance. *Performance skills,* the observable elements of action of an occupation, can be subdivided into motor and praxis, sensory–perceptual, cognitive processing, emotional regulatory, and communication and social skills.

Older adults with low vision may present with deficits in many of these performance skills. For example, motor skills may be compromised as the result of a low vision diagnosis because reaching for items becomes difficult when the client cannot clearly see the item for which he or she is reaching. Balance in the shower or during nighttime ambulation to the bathroom may become problematic when the client cannot clearly recognize his or her surroundings. Additionally, when considering the use of low vision devices (LVDs), it is important

that the occupational therapist assess whether the client has the coordination skills and sensory–perceptual skills to manipulate the device and the cognitive skills to understand its proper use. If LVDs are not recommended, the occupational therapist must evaluate whether the client has the necessary hearing or tactile sensation to use auditory or tactile strategies.

Remembering that vision loss can cause physical and psychosocial challenges and be accompanied by various age-related comorbid conditions is also important. During the early phases of adjustment to the visual impairment, the client may not be ready to address the functional implications of the vision loss and may deny the permanence or seriousness of the visual impairment or become angry or depressed. All practitioners working with people with visual impairment must understand and address the psychosocial issues associated with visual loss.

People with visual impairment are at increased risk—as high as 32.5%—of developing depression, emotional distress, and a reduction in quality of life (Rovner, Casten & Tasman, 2002; Slakter & Stur, 2005). Age-related vision loss often is progressive, although the rate of progression varies greatly among people. People with vision loss can experience feelings of depression, loss of control, dependency, and loss of role or identity (Brody et al., 2002; Mangione, Gutierrez, Lowe, Orav, & Seddon, 1999; Rovner et al., 2002; Scott, Schein, Feuer, Folstein, & Bandeen-Roche, 2001; Teitelman & Copolillo, 2005; Williams, Brody, Thomas, Kaplan, & Brown, 1998). How quickly one loses vision or the severity of the vision loss may threaten to impede occupational performance, but it does not predict a person's well-being, because people respond differently to loss (Horowitz & Reinhardt, 2000). People who accept their vision loss are more likely to use adaptations and compensatory strategies, thereby leading to participation in valued occupations (Teitelman & Copolillo, 2005). Screening for depression using tools such as the Geriatric Depression Scale (Yesavage et al., 1982–1983),

Box 3. Case Study: Analysis of Occupational Performance

A comprehensive occupational therapy assessment was completed with **Lillian**.

Canadian Occupational Performance Measure (COPM) Results:

Performance Area	Importance	Performance	Satisfaction
Self-care Personal care: Medication management	10	3	2
Self-care Community management: Finances	7	2	3
Productivity Household management: Cooking	9	2	3
Leisure Quiet recreation: Reading	9	2	1

COPM Performance Score 1: 9/4 = 2.25
COPM Satisfaction Score 1: 9/4 = 2.25

Eccentric Viewing and Preferred Retinal Locus: When mapping the scotomas using the clock method, Lillian's eccentric viewing position was found to be at 2 o'clock.

Reading & Writing: Tools used to assess reading and writing skills included the MNRead, the Collins Low Vision Writing Assessment, and the Pepper Visual Skills for Reading Test (VSRT).

MNRead: Critical print size 2 M at 80 words/minute.

Collins Low Vision Writing Assessment:

Writing grocery list	7/10
Writing recording checks	8/10
Written language	7/10
Reading notes to self	7/10
Completing a form	7/10
Total score:	36/50

Pepper VSRT:
Accuracy score: 80%
Words/minute: 70
Errors: Misidentification, omissions to right

the Center for Epidemiological Studies Depression Scale (Radloff, 1977), or the Patient Health Questionnaire (Spitzer, Kroenke, & Williams, 1999) can be a valuable method of evaluating depressive symptoms in people with vision loss.

Communication skills often are affected by low vision because reading and writing tasks are difficult to perform with limited visual acuity or visual field. A central scotoma or reduced visual acuity may lead to errors in reading financial statements, medication labels, and other important information. Reduced vision can make writing legibly difficult. Difficulty with performance skills such as making eye contact, recognizing faces, or interpreting nonverbal cues may negatively affect socialization. Additionally, low vision can lead to feelings of depression, so monitoring a client's emotional status is also important.

Several standard assessments are available to measure the performance skills of an older adult with low vision, as outlined in Table 2. Specifically, assessments of reading and writing can be used to gain objective information about an older adult's ability to perform these skills in a timely, accurate, and legible manner. The MNRead Acuity Charts (Mansfield et al., 1994) use a continuous-text reading format rather than the letter or symbol identification format of traditional acuity charts. They include 19 sentences, each in a different type size, all 60 characters in length, which are read from a 40-cm distance. The MNRead measures both acuity level and reading speed while at the same time identifying the smallest type size at which a person can read at his or her maximum speed (Mansfield et al., 1994). The MNRead charts have demonstrated reliability (Patel, Chen, Da Cruz, Rubin, & Tufail, 2011; Subramanian & Pardhan, 2006).

Another useful measure of reading performance, specifically for people with central field impairment, is the Pepper Visual Skills for Reading Test (VSRT), also known as the Pepper Test (Watson et al., 1995). It is a 10- to 15-minute assessment of the visual skills needed for reading and includes scores for reading accuracy and reading speed (Watson et al., 1995). Test materials are in five different type sizes ranging from newspaper print to newspaper headline print, and three equivalent forms of the test allow for retesting (Watson et al., 1995). The test administrator records the amount of time it takes to complete the test as well as the errors that occur during the test. Both reliability and validity testing have been completed and have demonstrated that the VSRT is a useful

assessment of reading for people with low vision (Baldasare, Watson, Whittaker, & Miller-Shaffer, 1986; Watson, Baldasare, & Whittaker, 1990; Watson et al., 1995).

Similarly, the Morgan Low Vision Reading Comprehension Assessment (LVRCA) is used to assess the reading comprehension of people with AMD to determine reading level (Watson, Wright, & Long, 1996). It includes 10 reading cards printed in 1 M, 1.5 M, 2 M, and 3 M font size at reading levels from 2nd to 12th grade. The LVRCA is an untimed test that uses the cloze method to determine reading comprehension. In the cloze method, a word in a sentence is replaced with a line; the individual is then asked to supply a word using the context of the sentence. The results can be used to assist the therapist in determining appropriate reading materials. Both reliability and validity testing have been established and demonstrated that the LVRCA is a useful assessment of reading comprehension for adults with AMD (Watson, Wright, Long, & De l'Aune, 1996).

In addition to reading skills, older adults with low vision often experience difficulties in writing tasks. A person needs to visually follow the hand—specifically, the pen tip and the writing on the page—to ensure that writing is legible (Watson, Wright, et al., 2004). Because writing is critical for the performance of many occupations, specifically assessing this performance skill is important. The Low Vision Writing Assessment formally addresses writing for older adults with low vision. It can be administered in 10–15 minutes in a variety of settings, including the home or clinic (Watson, Wright, et al., 2004). The assessment includes five tasks that represent typical writing necessary in everyday life that often becomes difficult for older adults with low vision. The tasks include writing a grocery list, writing a check and updating the account register, writing a prose paragraph, filling out a health information form, and reading aloud the grocery list composed during the assessment. It can be used to gather baseline data as well as to measure progress after intervention and has established reliability and validity (Watson, Wright, et al., 2004).

Client Factors

Client factors are the underlying abilities, values, beliefs, and spirituality; body functions; and body structures that affect the person's occupational performance. The client factors discussed here as they pertain to older adults with low vision include visual function adjustment to the visual loss and mental and sensory function.

The occupational therapy practitioner assesses specific aspects of vision, including (1) visual function, (2) visual efficiency, and (3) visual perception. *Visual function* includes the basic visual skills of acuity (distance and near), contrast sensitivity, visual field, ocular motility, eye alignment, convergence, and accommodation. *Visual efficiency* includes attention to the object of regard, tracking skills, scanning, object discrimination, and ability to detect fine detail. Finally, *visual perception* includes higher level visual skills, including visual attention, visual scanning, pattern recognition, visual memory, and visual cognition. Occupational therapy practitioners understand the impact of these client factors on engagement in occupations.

Methods to assess these visual client factors are described in several occupational therapy resources (Quintana, 2008; Warren, 2006; Zoltan, 2007). Additionally, each of the factors listed in the preceding paragraph is included in the Brain Injury Visual Assessment Battery for Adults (biVABA; Warren, 1998), a comprehensive assessment of visual functioning that consists of several separate, individually developed screening tools. Many of the screening tools in the biVABA have been developed by professionals in ophthalmology and optometry and have undergone psychometric testing (Warren, 1998). The biVABA is organized according to Warren's (1993a, 1993b) visual–perceptual hierarchy, which places visual acuity (including contrast sensitivity), visual field, and oculomotor control at the foundation of that hierarchy pyramid.

Because these visual skills are foundational, impairment at this level causes difficulty in higher visual processing skills, including visual attention, scanning, pattern recognition, visual memory, and visuocognition (Warren, 1993a, 1993b). Therefore, assessment of visual acuity, visual field, and oculomotor control is an essential component of the evaluation of a person presenting with low vision. For examples of assessment tools, please refer to Table 2.

In addition to visual function, it is important that the occupational therapist assess the mental function of the person with low vision. Attention, memory, sequencing, problem solving, and judgment, among others, are critical cognitive skills that enable an older adult with low vision to adapt to vision loss. Therefore, an evaluation of these factors will enhance the overall evaluation of the older adult with low vision and will provide critical information to the occupational therapy practitioner that will be useful in intervention planning. The assessment of cognitive status can begin with screening tools such as the Mini-Mental State Examination (Folstein, Folstein, & McHugh, 1975) or the Montreal Cognitive Assessment (Nasreddine, 2011) and, if needed, can continue with a more in-depth assessment using tools such as the Loewenstein Occupational Therapy Cognitive Assessment (Itzkovish et al., 1990) or the Cognitive Assessment of Minnesota (Rustad et al., 1993).

Finally, sensory function also should be assessed as a part of the occupational therapy assessment for older adults with low vision. As with cognition, sensation plays a critical role in the adaptation to visual loss because tactile sensation and hearing can become substitutes in tasks that were once primarily done using the visual system. Therefore, knowledge about whether these systems are intact, impaired, or absent is an essential component of the overall assessment of an older adult with low vision.

Performance Patterns

Performance patterns are behaviors related to customary daily life activities (AOTA, 2008); they include habits, routines, rituals, and roles. These habits and routines can either be beneficial or interfere with occupational performance.

Older adults with low vision rely on habits and routines to remain independent. For example, a person may routinely place an item in a specific, reliable location, which allows the person to rely on his or her memory rather than vision to locate the item. This routine allows the person to remain independent and reduces the risk of frustration. In contrast, if a person completes his or her medication management at the kitchen table without an established organizational system, there is a risk of medication mismanagement. Evaluating a client's current performance patterns through interview and observing the client engaging in areas of occupation will allow the occupational therapy practitioner to understand those habits, routines, rituals, and roles that are beneficial to or interfere with occupational performance.

Contexts and Environment

Occupational therapy practitioners acknowledge the influence of cultural, personal, temporal, virtual, physical, and social contextual factors on occupations and activities. Environmental factors that support or hinder the occupational performance of older adults with low vision should be identified throughout the evaluation and intervention process. The number of standardized assessments that specifically address contexts for older adults with low vision is limited. Therefore, much of the evaluation of contexts is done in an informal manner.

Cultural

The cultural context includes the customs, beliefs, activity patterns, behavior standards, and expectations accepted by the client and his or her cultural group. Some of these patterns of performance (e.g., shaking hands when greeting someone, making eye contact when speaking with someone) may be difficult for older adults with low vision. Occupational therapy practitioners provide culturally responsive care by displaying an awareness of and sensitivity to the client's cultural beliefs about health and how culture may influence the client's typical activity patterns and occupations. By engaging in culturally competent care, the occupational therapist will incorporate the client's values, beliefs, ways of life, and practices into a mutually acceptable treatment plan.

Personal

Personal attributes such as gender, socioeconomic status, age, and level of education all factor into the evaluation and intervention process. Although this Practice Guideline is aimed at low vision rehabilitation in the older adult population, visual impairment can occur at any time in a person's life, so considering these personal contexts is important to provide culturally and age-appropriate assessment and interventions.

Socioeconomic status can affect assessment and intervention; for example, commonly recommended devices or adaptations for older adults with low vision are not reimbursed by most third-party payers and would thus be out-of-pocket expenses. It is important to understand the potential barriers to accessing services or recommended devices and either provide alternatives or advocate for the client to obtain the necessary services or devices.

Temporal

On a large scale, *temporal context* may refer to the time in a person's life course in which the vision loss may have occurred, such as adulthood or late adulthood. Temporal context also can refer to the stage of vision loss or onset, which influences decisions about choice of evaluation tools and treatment interventions because the stage of adjustment or readiness for assessment and intervention may vary. Age of onset also can affect assessment and intervention decision making; for example, a person with retinitis pigmentosa diagnosed with the condition at age 12 is now aging with a disability and may be dealing with challenges such as arthritis or diabetes. In this case, previous strategies for community mobility, such as use of a long cane, may now create challenges because of arthritic changes in the hand and wrist or peripheral neuropathy from diabetes.

Physical

The physical context is an important component of the evaluation of an older adult with low vision. The occupational therapist evaluates the physical environment for supports and barriers to the client's occupational performance. Evaluation of the client's home, workplace, and commonly used community locations is important to support engagement in occupational performance.

It is important to remember that assessment of the physical environment must take into consideration that this is an aging population. In addition to the traditional home and community assessment, components of the evaluation of the physical context should include the following:

- *Lighting:* With aging come changes to the eye that require increased lighting. The average older adult requires an illumination level that is 3–4 times brighter than that of a younger person (Figueiro, 2001). When evaluating lighting and lighting levels, one should consider the location of the light (Is it an ambient light or a task light?), the number and position of light fixtures, potential glare (windows, window coverings, and highly polished surfaces), the amount of contrast between the foreground and the background, and the quality of the light (Is the light uniform? What type of lighting is present?). A light meter is recommended to measure lighting levels accurately. Adequate ambient lighting

in the home is 300 to 500 lux, whereas task-specific lighting should be at least 1,000 lux (Boyce & Sanford, 2000; Figueiro, 2001). The forthcoming Home Environment Lighting Assessment (Perlmutter, n.d.) may be useful in accurately assessing lighting on the basis of the functional activities that the client performs in various locations throughout the home.

- *Contrast:* Similar to assessment of lighting, assessment of the contrast in the client's environment should be a major consideration when evaluating the physical environment. For example, a typical bathroom may have white walls, white floors, a white bathtub, a white toilet, white towels, and white adaptive equipment, which makes it difficult for the older adult with low vision to distinguish one from another. Locating the bath bench inside the bathtub or the edge of the tub in contrast to the floor and the walls can become problematic. Likewise, in the kitchen, an older adult with low vision may have difficulty locating and using the dial on the stove or microwave or reading the ingredients on food packaging.

- *Organization:* The occupational therapist should assess the presence or absence of organizational strategies as part of the assessment of the physical environment of an older adult with low vision. Observation is one method the occupational therapist can use to identify the level of organization throughout the home environment. For example, observation of the organizational strategies used in kitchen cupboards, bedroom closets, or bathroom drawers can provide useful information in understanding the types of strategies the older adult with low vision has already implemented. If observation of the physical environment is not practical, the older adult with low vision may provide a self-report of the types of strategies that he or she may or may not be using throughout the home to assist him or her in performing daily occupations.

Occupational therapists' knowledge of the influence of the environment on occupational performance makes them well suited to assess the environment.

Social

The social environment or context includes the social network of friends, family, groups, and organizations with whom the client has contact. These social relationships carry expectations for interaction, and the older adult with low vision may be challenged when functioning within the social environment. Difficulty following the pragmatics or interaction rules of social environments (e.g., an inability to read nonverbal communication, not being able to recognize people's faces in a social environment) can contribute to social isolation. Some clients may have drifted away from family and friends because they have struggled to remain in their social roles (e.g., they may have discontinued bingo or card groups because of an inability to read the cards or discontinued lunch group because of difficulty reading menus or fear of falling).

Virtual

The virtual environment is one in which communication occurs by means of airways or computers and an absence of physical contact. Assistive technologies, such as screen readers, voice recognition telephones, or books on tape or compact disc, can be used to compensate for vision loss in support of occupational performance (Jutai, Strong, & Russell-Minda, 2009). Occupational therapists may need to evaluate the client's previous use of technology to interact in the virtual environment (e.g., use of and expertise in e-mailing and text messaging, conversing in chat rooms). The client's level of comfort with the tools of the virtual environment may guide the occupational therapist in selecting possible assistive technology (e.g., ZoomText Screen Magnifier/Reader by Ai Squared, Manchester Center, VT; JAWS Screen Reading Software by Freedom Scientific, St. Petersbury, FL; Dragon Naturally Speaking by Nuance Communications, Burlington, MA) during the intervention phase.

Activity Demands

Determining whether a client may be able to complete an activity depends not only on the person's performance skills, performance patterns, and client factors but also on the demands the activity itself places on the person. The demands of an activity include the tools needed to carry out the activity, the space and social demands required by the activity, and the required actions and performance skills needed to take part in the given activity.

Many older adults with low vision must use LVDs (microscopes, hand and stand magnifiers, telescopes), assistive technology (electronic magnification, computer software), or both to complete ADLs and IADLs. Figure 4 illustrates a variety of LVDs and assistive technology for completion of occupations. These devices require the individual to understand how the device is used; to have the motor control, strength, and endurance to manipulate the device; and to have adequate visual function to use the device.

In addition, because of LVD, lighting, and other demands, having a specific environment established for a specific task is often necessary. For example, a reading and writing area may need to be established that allows for adequate lighting (a gooseneck table lamp positioned on the work surface), proper positioning (flat surface allowing the stand magnifier to be held flat on the reading surface), and suitable space to allow for successful task completion.

Considerations in Assessment

Most occupational therapy practitioners do not specialize in low vision but experience the impact of vision loss as a result of secondary conditions on their clients' occupational performance. A person has a primary diagnosis of low vision when a health condition, such as AMD, is causing the visual impairment. Conversely, a person has a secondary diagnosis of low vision when a health

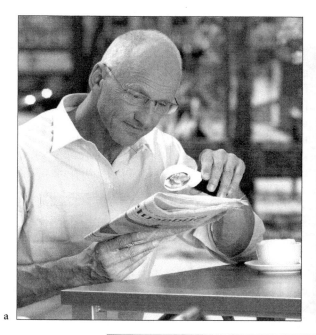
a

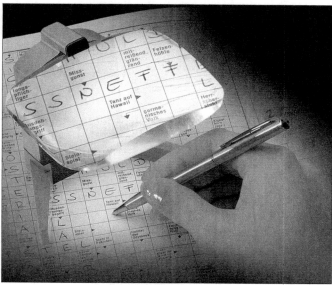
b

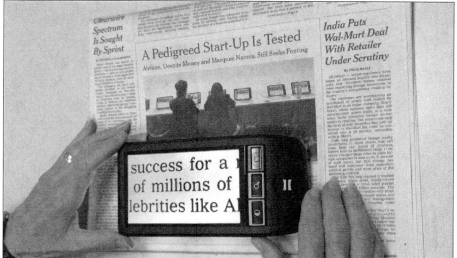
c

Figure 4. Low vision devices and assistive technology: (a) handheld magnifier used for reading newsprint, (b) stand magnifier used for completing a crossword puzzle, and (c) portable closed-circuit television used for reading the newspaper.

condition, such as long-term diabetes leading to diabetic retinopathy, causes the visual impairment (in addition to other potential secondary diagnoses such as peripheral neuropathy).

Intervention strategies that may be effective with one older adult with low vision, such as using tactile markings for object identification, may not be helpful for another older adult with multiple impairments, such as a decreased visual field combined with peripheral neuropathy. Therefore, it is important to keep in mind the underlying pathology of the low vision diagnosis.

In addition, older adults often present with several concurrent health conditions that can have an impact on their ability to participate in occupations of choice but also have an impact on assessment and intervention. It is important to be aware of and understand the impact of comorbidities, secondary conditions, and associated conditions on the person and his or her occupational performance. For example, in working with a person who has AMD as well as Parkinson's disease and moderate dementia, understanding the primary diagnosis and the concurrent conditions may affect the occupational therapist's clinical reasoning in determining assessment and intervention strategies. Given that tremor is associated with Parkinson's disease, handheld LVDs would be avoided or, knowing that new learning is more difficult for people with dementia, the therapist may choose environmental modifications rather than electronic magnification.

As a result of binocular visual deficits, impaired depth perception, visual field defects, general decline in visual acuity, and reduced contrast sensitivity, people with visual impairment are at increased risk for mobility and balance deficits as well as for falls (Coleman et al., 2004; Ivers, Cumming, Mitchell, Simpson, & Peduto, 2003; Lee & Scudds, 2003; Lord & Dayhew, 2001). General assessments of balance and coordination that are used in other areas of occupational therapy practice can be used with this population to better quantify the client's safety with tasks involving these client factors (refer to Table 2).

In addition to safety, it is also important to understand how vision affects a person's quality of life. Additional assessment tools can be used to measure vision-related quality of life (Mangione et al., 2001; Wolffsohn & Cochrane, 2000). The Low Vision Quality-of-Life Questionnaire is a 25-item self-report measure designed to identify quality-of-life issues associated with permanent visual impairment as well as to measure the effectiveness of low vision rehabilitation on quality of life (Wolffsohn & Cochrane, 2000). Similarly, the 25-item National Eye Institute Visual Function Questionnaire also was developed to measure vision-related quality of life (Mangione et al., 2001). It is a shorter version of the original 51-item assessment designed to be more useful for administration in clinical settings because of its shorter length and is intended to be administered in an interview format (Mangione et al., 2001). Both of these assessments have undergone reliability and validity testing and have proven to be appropriate tools for use in the clinical setting (Mangione et al., 2001; Wolffsohn & Cochrane, 2000).

It is critical that therapists use their knowledge of assessments and clinical judgment to decide which assessments should be selected for each client at a particular time. This careful selection of assessments provides the most valuable data and eliminates the tendency to bombard the client with excessive assessment demands. Understanding the typical course and prognosis of the ocular condition and the typical impact on occupational performance can help the occupational therapist determine when it is most appropriate to focus on various components of the client's occupational performance and the types of assessments to administer.

Intervention

Occupational therapy intervention for older adults with low vision may occur throughout the course of the low vision diagnosis as needs change. The intervention, guided by information about the client gathered during the evaluation, incorporates a variety of approaches using preparatory methods (i.e., therapist-selected methods and techniques that prepare the client for occupational performance, such as eccentric viewing training or scanning exercises), purposeful interventions (i.e., specifically selected activities that allow the client to develop skills that enhance occupational engagement, such as role-playing of social situations or practicing grocery shopping in a simulated environment), and occupation-based interventions (i.e., client-directed occupations in context that match identified goals, such as reading letters or financial statements with an optical device or writing a grocery list using strategies that enhance readability). The focus of intervention may shift among establishing, restoring, or maintaining occupational performance; modifying the environment or contexts and activity demands or patterns; promoting health; or preventing further disability and occupational performance problems.

Intervention Plan

As a part of the occupational therapy process, the occupational therapist develops an intervention plan that considers the client's goals, values, and beliefs; the client's health and well-being; the client's performance skills and performance patterns; collective influence of the context, environment, activity demands, and client factors on the client's performance; and the context of service delivery in which the intervention is provided (e.g., caregiver expectations, organization's purpose, payer's requirements, applicable regulations; AOTA, 2008). The intervention plan outlines and guides the therapist's actions and is based on the best available evidence to meet the identified outcomes.

Once the therapist has identified targeted goals in collaboration with the client or family, the therapist determines the intervention approach that is best suited to address these goals. Some approaches may be more appropriate at various times than others. The intervention approaches used by occupational therapy practitioners include the following:

- *Prevent,* an intervention approach designed to address clients with or without disability who are at risk for occupational performance problems (Dunn, McClain, Brown, & Youngstrom, 1998), for example, intervention to prevent falls because people with visual impairment are at increased risk of falls;
- *Establish and restore,* an intervention approach designed to change client variables to establish a skill or ability that has not yet developed or to restore a skill or ability that has been impaired (Dunn et al., 1998); for this population, the occupational therapy practitioner needs to carefully

distinguish between establishing a new skill and restoring an ability that has been impaired (e.g., a person can establish a new skill such as eccentric viewing, but it should not be confused with the restoration of the visual function);
- *Modify activity demands and the contexts,* an approach in which activities are performed to support safe, independent performance of valued activities within the constraints of motor, cognitive, or perceptual limitations; for example, modifying the home environment with increased lighting, color contrast, and reduction of clutter;
- *Create or promote a healthy and satisfying lifestyle,* an approach that includes adherence to medication routine, appropriate diet, appropriate levels of physical activity, and satisfying levels of engagement in social relationships and activities by providing enriched contextual and activity experiences that will enhance performance for all people in the natural contexts of life (Dunn et al., 1998); for example, teaching a client to consistently use sun protection, such as filters or a wide-brimmed hat; and
- *Maintain performance and health,* an approach used with the older adult with low vision, for example, ensuring that an older adult who has diabetic retinopathy can accurately perform medication management.

Occupational therapy practitioners also consider the types of interventions when determining the most effective treatment plan for a given client. The types of interventions include therapeutic use of self; therapeutic use of occupations and activities, which includes preparatory methods, purposeful activity, and occupation-based activity; consultation; and education. Although all types of occupational therapy interventions are used for all approaches, the therapeutic use of self (i.e., therapist's use of his or her personality, perception, and judgment; AOTA, 2008) is an overarching concept that should be considered during each therapeutic interaction. Therapeutic use of self is a vital responsibility of the occupational therapist and occupational therapy assistant, as well as of all members of the health care team.

Best Practices and Summaries of Evidence

The following sections include both an overview of specific interventions and findings from the systematic reviews of occupational therapy for older adults with low vision. A standard process of searching for and reviewing literature related to practice with older adults with low vision was used, and this process is summarized in Appendix C. The research studies presented here include primarily *Level I* randomized controlled trials; *Level II* studies, in which assignment to a treatment or a control group is not randomized (cohort study); and *Level III* studies, which do not have a control group. In this systematic review, evidence for occupational therapy practice from studies at Levels I, II, and III was used to answer a particular question. All studies identified by the review, including those not specifically described in this section, are summarized and cited in full in the evidence tables in Appendix D. Readers are encouraged to read the full articles for more details.

For each area of intervention, consistent results in two or more Level I studies were considered as strong evidence, and consistent results in one Level I study plus more than two lower-level studies were considered as moderate evidence (U.S. Preventive Services Task Force, 2008). When only one Level I study or consistent results in multiple lower level studies were found, these interventions were rated as having limited evidence (U.S. Preventive Services Task Force, 2008). Finally, inconsistent results between studies were described as having mixed evidence.

Intervention Implementation

Currently, vision that has been lost as the result of AMD, diabetic retinopathy, or glaucoma cannot be restored. Therefore, the goal of low vision rehabilitation is to teach the client ways to compensate for the visual deficit to increase the ability to complete daily tasks independently by altering the task through the use of adaptive equipment, strategies, LVDs, or assistive technology; modifying the environment through increased lighting and environmental modifications; or adapting the person's capabilities through scotoma awareness training and eccentric viewing training.

To compensate for vision loss and continue to engage in occupations of choice, older adults with low vision first must acknowledge the permanence of their visual impairment and identify areas of occupation that are affected by the vision loss. As a result of perceptual completion, or the brain's tendency to automatically fill in any missing information with what it thinks should be there, some older adults with low vision may not fully realize that they have a visual impairment. Without awareness of a visual impairment, the client cannot understand or realize the benefits of intervention, and therefore adherence to a rehabilitation plan would be mixed. Consequently, education is essential throughout the rehabilitation process. It is important that the client and his or her family understand the nature of the ocular disease or condition, its prognosis, and the associated symptoms. In addition, throughout the rehabilitation process, the client needs to be educated on the intervention strategies that may facilitate engagement in desired occupations. Through the provision of ongoing education and instruction in active problem solving, people can gain a sense of control over their circumstances (Dahlin Ivanoff, Sonn, & Svensson, 2002; Rovner & Casten, 2008).

Once an older adult with low vision has a clear understanding that a visual impairment exists, he or she can use several strategies to compensate for the impairment. These strategies may include the following:

- Developing visual skills such as the use of eccentric viewing or a preferred retinal locus (PRL) or scanning strategies
- Training in the use of optical or electronic magnification devices; assistive technology
- Training in use of nonoptical strategies
- Using sensory substitution strategies (tactile and auditory)
- Maximizing organizational strategies
- Modifying the environment
- Training in appropriate community mobility strategies
- Learning active problem solving
- Advocating for needed assistive technology, environmental modifications, or other services
- Training in the use of community resources
- Referral
- Routines and habits.

Each of these strategies is discussed separately; however, it is important to understand that several of these strategies are used in combination to create a comprehensive plan to maximize the client's ability to participate in valued occupations throughout the day. It is also important to remember that many of these strategies also could be considered cognitive strategies because they require the client to use components of cognition such as problem solving, recall, sequencing, memory, and judgment.

Visual Skills Training

Older adults with either peripheral or central visual field impairment can learn techniques to maximize awareness of their visual field. For peripheral visual field loss, an organized method of visual scanning can be taught to improve attention and responsiveness to the environment and to increase safety. An organized scanning pattern such as left to right, top to bottom, or the use of anchoring (i.e., a visual cue to the starting position or to the left margin of a page) can be helpful for reading and functional tasks. In addition, incorporating sensorimotor activities during scanning tasks, within the context of the task (i.e., reaching for canned goods in a pantry as the person scans the shelves), can facilitate greater carryover (Quintana, 2008; Warren, 1993b).

For central visual field loss, training in eccentric viewing can allow the older adult to use an alternate viewing area or PRL to maximize use of residual vision. Eccentric viewing begins with the older adult becoming aware of the scotoma. The scotomas can be mapped, using the face of a clock (refer to Figure 5). Once the scotoma has been identified, mapped, and understood, the older adult can be trained to move the scotoma out of the way by looking in the direction of the scotoma, which allows healthier retinal tissue to perceive the object of regard. Eccentric viewing, or use of the PRL, can be used for distance and near tasks. Note that cognitive impairment or client preference may be a limiting factor for using eccentric viewing as an intervention strategy.

According to Schuchard (2005), the goal of eccentric viewing training is to enable a person who has a central scotoma to use another area of the retina (a PRL) as a focal point. He noted that many people who have central scotomas are unaware that the blind spot even exists. Therefore, he concluded that education in the awareness of the scotomas is valuable if only for the purpose of increased insight into the visual impairment. He stated that people who are aware of their scotomas are "more likely to make more accurate compensatory eye movements to search for, find, and identify pertinent visual information" (p. 309).

Although most of the research on eccentric viewing and the PRL has been cross-sectional in nature,

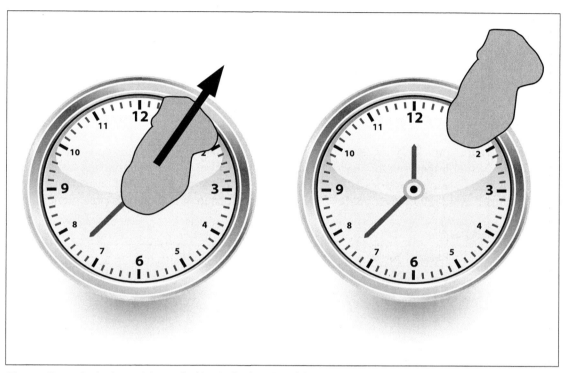

Figure 5. Eccentric viewing training. By looking in the direction of the scotoma (arrow), the scotoma is moved out of the way.

Crossland, Culham, Kabanarou, and Rubin (2005) performed a longitudinal study of the development of the PRL in people with macular degeneration. They determined that people who have bilateral central scotomas naturally develop a PRL within 6 months, and many of them develop not only one PRL but several of them. Interestingly, Crossland and colleagues also found that people who were unaware of eccentric viewing strategies actually performed better in reading speed than people who were aware that they were using a PRL instead of their fovea. Therefore, when a PRL is used automatically without conscious awareness of it, reading performance is often improved.

Summary of the Evidence to Support Visual Skills Training

In the systematic review regarding visual skills training, four studies examined the effects of training in specialized viewing techniques, including eccentric viewing and binocular or monocular viewing, on reading performance of older adults with AMD (Frennesson, Jakobsson, & Nilsson, 1995; Kabanarou & Rubin, 2006; Vukicevic & Fitzmaurice, 2005, 2009). Kabanarou and Rubin (2006) and Vukicevic and Fitzmaurice (2005) provided Level I evidence, whereas Vukicevic and Fitzmaurice (2009) provided Level II evidence and Frennesson and colleagues (1995) provided Level III evidence. These studies found limited evidence supporting eccentric viewing completed with specific computer software programs for near vision and ADLs. In addition, the evidence to support eccentric viewing in combination with instruction in magnification is limited (Vukicevic & Fitzmaurice, 2005). Kabanarou and Rubin (2006) compared the effects of binocular and monocular viewing and found no evidence supporting one technique over the other. Because of the small sample sizes in several of these studies, higher quality research is needed to substantiate the implementation of eccentric viewing training and other viewing techniques for people with AMD and central scotomas.

Magnification

Magnification devices are commonly prescribed for older adults with visual impairment to assist with completion of near, intermediate, or distance tasks. Although some commercially available large-print books are viable solutions for some older adults with low vision, for others the amount of enlargement is not sufficient to enable a return to their prior activities and pastimes.

Many types of magnification or LVDs are available: microscopes (high plus spectacles), stand magnifiers, handheld magnifiers, telescopes, and electronic magnification. Each device has its own pros and cons, which must be considered in determining best fit between the individual, the device, and the activity being performed, as can be seen in Table 3. The occupational therapy practitioner must ensure

Table 3. Types of Low Vision Devices

Type of Device	Range of Power	Pros	Cons
Microscopes (high plus spectacles)	• Binocular, $+1.00$ D to $+14$ D • Monocular, ≤ 64 D	• Relatively inexpensive • Commonly accepted • In low powers, cosmetically appealing and allows for a wide field of view • Portable	• In high powers, focal distance is reduced.
Stand magnifier (convex lens that is set to be held at its focal distance)	• 6 D to 50+ D	• Because it is set at its focal distance, does not have to be held • Allows for a greater focal distance • Inexpensive	• Because of its size, it is not as portable as a hand-held magnifier. • In nonilluminated forms, there is less light because of the housing. • Must ensure proper ergonomics because the device must be held flat; individuals often lean over to view.
Hand magnifier (convex lens with a handle that the individual must hold at the focal distance of the lens)	• 2 D to 50+ D	• Good for spotting tasks • Portable • Inexpensive	• Focal distance must be maintained by the individual (eye to lens and lens to object).
Telescopes (Galilean or Keplarian; monocular or binocular)	• 0.5× to 20×	• Good for distance spotting • Can be modified for near and intermediate tasks • In a low power, can be used in reverse for field awareness	• Limited field of view • Limited depth of focus
Electronic magnification (closed-circuit television)	• Up to 70× magnification	• Good for extended reading, writing, and leisure activities • Large range of power • Can modify lighting and contrast • Wide field of view • Comes in tabletop and portable versions	• Expensive • Portability • Requires more training than other devices

Note. D = *diopter,* a unit measure of refractive power of a lens.

proper ergonomics with optical and electronic magnification devices because proper positioning has been shown to increase reading speed and improve comfort with reading tasks (Watson, Ramsey, De l'Aune, & Elk, 2004).

Several research teams have found that older adults with low vision who use electronic magnification showed greater improvements in reading speed and duration than when using other types of optical devices (Goodrich & Kirby, 2001; Goodrich, Kirby, Wagstaff, Oros, & McDevitt, 2004; Peterson, Wolffsohn, Rubinstein, & Lowe, 2003; Stelmack, Reda, Ahlers, Bainbridge, & McCray, 1991); however, not all activities can be completed with electronic magnification systems, and for some people, electronic magnification is cost prohibitive. Thus, electronic magnification systems are not accessible to everyone.

McIlwaine, Bell, and Dutton (1991) studied the use of low vision aids among people with low vision. They determined that approximately one-third of the low vision aids that were being dispensed through a low vision clinic were not being used and that one-half of the clients who had the devices were not satisfied with them. As they compared their service provision with that of other low vision programs, they concluded that other programs had a much higher success rate in low vision aid use because the clients of those clinics also received several training sessions in the use of the low vision aids and follow-up home visits if needed (McIlwaine et al., 1991).

These findings are consistent with those of Humphry and Thompson (1986), who found that the success rate of device use was only 23% for those who did not receive training in proper use of the device. Therefore, research has suggested that the success rate of low vision aids to improve visual ability is greater when those who are prescribed the devices also are trained in their proper use.

Fok, Polgar, Shaw, and Jutai (2011) studied low vision aid usage and reasons for device abandonment and found that approximately 30% of all low vision aids are left unused or abandoned.

Device abandonment was found to be related to (1) lack of consideration of client needs when considering devices; (2) difficulty in device use or a poor fit between the device and client factors; (3) poor device performance or devices did not match the client's needs or goals; (4) financial, physical, or psychological accessibility of the device; and (5) a lack of perceived need for the LVD (Fok et al., 2011; Mann, Goodall, Justiss, & Tomita, 2002; Phillips & Zhao, 1993; Riemer-Reiss & Wacker, 2000). Additionally, they found that when devices were accepted by the client and used appropriately, they were helpful in facilitating participation in occupations of choice.

After a comprehensive low vision examination by the eye care professional, the occupational therapist and eye care professional collaborate to determine the best magnification strategies. No single device will meet the needs of all older adults with low vision and all potential occupations. If optical devices are determined to be the best solution, they are prescribed by the eye care professional. Then the occupational therapy practitioner can teach the client how to effectively use them, taking into consideration the client's needs and abilities.

Summary of the Evidence to Support Magnification

In the systematic review, five studies supplying Level II and Level III evidence examined the effectiveness of LVDs in improving reading performance (Bowers, Lovie-Kitchin, & Woods, 2001; Cheong, Lovie-Kitchin, Bowers, & Brown, 2005; Horowitz, Brennan, Reinhardt, & Macmillan, 2006; Margrain, 2000; Nguyen, Weismann, & Trauzettel-Klosinski, 2009). The types of LVDs included in the studies consisted of high-add spectacles, nonilluminated and illuminated hand-held magnifiers, nonilluminated and illuminated stand magnifiers, high plus lenses, telescopes, and electronic magnifiers such as CCTVs. Margrain (2000) and Nguyen and colleagues (2009) compared participants' ability to read before and after the introduction of

LVDs. Both research groups found a significant difference in the number of participants able to read with a device as opposed to without it.

Horowitz and colleagues (2006) found that the use of optical devices decreases the level of disability when performing ADLs. Finally, Bowers, Lovie-Kitchin, and Woods (2001) and Cheong and colleagues (2005) studied the difference between reading at critical print size with and without an optical magnifier. They found that the use of a magnifier did not produce slower reading speeds as expected compared with reading at critical print size with no device.

Although all of these studies found that LVDs either improved reading speed or decreased the level of disability in performing IADLs, in combination they provided limited evidence to support the effectiveness of LVDs over no device use because the research designs lacked control groups and randomization. Therefore, more evidence of higher methodological quality is needed to determine the impact of LVDs on reading performance.

Five additional studies in the systematic review compared the effectiveness of optical and electronic magnifying devices on improving reading performance (Culham, Chabra, & Rubin, 2004; Goodrich & Kirby, 2001; Goodrich et al., 2004; Peterson et al., 2003; Stelmack et al., 1991). Of these studies, Goodrich and Kirby (2001) and Peterson and colleagues (2003) provided Level I evidence, and Goodrich and colleagues (2004), Culham and colleagues (2004), and Stelmack and colleagues (1991) provided Level II evidence. The types of LVDs in these studies include hand-held, stand-based, mouse-based, and head-mounted electronic magnification systems (also known as CCTVs; Culham et al., 2004; Goodrich & Kirby, 2001; Goodrich et al., 2004; Peterson et al., 2003; Stelmack et al., 1991); spectacle reading glasses (Culham et al., 2004; Stelmack et al., 1991); illuminated stand magnifiers (Stelmack et al., 1991); and the Nomad, which is an augmented reality system that projects an image directly on the retina using a laser (Goodrich et al., 2004).

Although each research group studied different combinations of optical and electronic devices, four of them concluded that use of stand-based electronic magnification systems produced faster reading rates (Goodrich & Kirby, 2001; Goodrich et al., 2004; Peterson et al., 2003; Stelmack et al., 1991) and longer reading duration (Goodrich & Kirby, 2001; Goodrich et al., 2004; Stelmack et al., 1991) than other devices. Therefore, the evidence for the use of stand-based electronic magnification systems is moderate. The evidence that hand-held electronic magnification is more beneficial than a prescribed optical device for reading purposes is limited (Goodrich & Kirby, 2001). Additionally, two of the studies (Culham et al., 2004; Stelmack et al., 1991) found mixed results regarding the effectiveness of spectacle reading glasses. Moreover, Culham and colleagues (2004, Level II) found that head-mounted electronic magnification systems are less effective than optical magnifiers for maximizing reading speed.

Sensory Substitution Strategies

As vision declines, older adults may begin to use alternative senses to compensate for the loss of visual input (Sokol-McKay, Buskirk, & Whittaker, 2003; Warren & Lampert, 1994). Older adults may use compensatory techniques, including auditory notifications to alert them to needed information or tactile presentation of information typically presented visually, to complete daily occupations. For example, tactile markings on appliance dials, pantry items, and toiletries can aid older adults with low vision in getting through their daily routines efficiently and accurately. Note, however, that people with diabetic retinopathy also may have tactile sensory impairments as a result of complications of neuropathy that may make compensation through the sense of touch difficult (Keeffe, Lam, Cheung, Dinh, & McCarty, 1998).

The aging eye has a reduced ability to detect short wavelengths, or "blue light," because of the yellowing of the lens (Figueiro, 2001). As a result, distinguishing blue from black may be difficult for older adults, regardless of their visual status. This decline tends to be most problematic when selecting and matching clothing. Attaching nonrusting safety pins to clothing labels in a systematic manner, such as one pin for blue clothes and two pins for black, enables older adults with low vision to identify colors through touch.

If an older adult is unable to use his or her visual or tactile senses, he or she can use auditory strategies to compensate for decreasing vision. Many talking products are commercially available, such as watches, clocks, scales, thermostats, and glucometers. In addition, free services are available to people with visual impairment who cannot access print, including books on tape or compact disc, telephone directory services, and newspaper reading services that promote engagement in these occupations.

Summary of the Evidence to Support Sensory Substitution Strategies

At the time of this review, no evidence on the effectiveness of sensory substitution strategies to compensate for vision loss met the inclusion criteria of the systematic review.

Organizational Strategies

When people cannot rely on their vision to easily and reliably locate items, organizational strategies can be helpful. Avoiding clutter, developing a regular cleaning schedule, and working with family and care providers to ensure reliable organization of items can improve safety and independence. For example, because clutter increases the risk of falls, eliminating unnecessary items in walkways and frequently used locations of the home can facilitate a safer environment. Clutter also can make it difficult to locate items, so determining a home location for items and reducing the number of superfluous items is a beneficial organizational strategy. If a person cannot locate his or her keys

on a table filled with mail, then consistently placing the keys on a hook by the door can increase efficiency and safety and decrease frustration.

Additionally, establishing a regular cleaning schedule can ensure a safer environment. For example, cleaning out the refrigerator on a biweekly basis and throwing out all dairy products ensures that spoiled foods will not be ingested unknowingly. Cleaning the floors first in one direction and then again in the opposite direction ensures that the entire surface is covered.

Finally, instructional sessions with family and caregivers can assist them in maintaining organizational strategies. For example, if the older adult completes his or her morning medication management in the kitchen and evening medication management at bedside, then maintaining an organized location with all necessary items can help ensure medication adherence. When an older adult with low vision is living with a spouse or others, those in the household must understand the importance of eliminating clutter and returning items to their home locations to increase independence and reduce frustration for the person with low vision.

Summary of the Evidence to Support Organizational Strategies

At the time of this review, no evidence on the effectiveness of organizational strategies to compensate for vision loss met the inclusion criteria of the systematic review.

Environmental Adaptations

Lighting Strategies and Summary of the Evidence to Support Lighting Strategies

As people age, normative changes in the eye occur that require increased lighting to resolve an image. A smaller pupil, changes to the cornea, and yellowing of the lens create the need for double or triple the amount of light needed by a younger person (Figueiro, 2001). Increased lighting has been shown to improve functional independence and quality of life for older adults with visual impairments (Brunnström, Sörensen, Alsterstad, & Sjöstrand, 2004). Increasing the amount of lighting for older adults and especially for older adults with low vision is a simple intervention to facilitate engagement in occupations of choice.

Ambient lighting supports safe mobility. Proper illumination can help highlight or identify obstacles in walkways and alert the older adult to changes in surface or conditions, such as walking from sidewalk to curb or tile to carpet. In addition, normative aging increases the time required for the eye to adapt when moving from a light to a dark environment. Therefore, both home and community environments should accommodate even illumination transitions between and within these spaces (Figueiro, 2001).

Task lighting supports near tasks, such as reading and writing, as well as social participation and ADLs (Bowers, Meek, & Stewart, 2001; Brunnström et al., 2004; Eldred, 1992; Eperjesi, Maiz-Fernandez, & Bartlett, 2007; Fosse & Valberg, 2004; Haymes & Lee, 2006). The use of a gooseneck table lamp or floor lamp is optimal for task lighting because it is flexible and can be adjusted to direct light onto the task rather than into the person's eyes. For reading tasks, positioning the light over the shoulder of the better seeing eye and directed onto the task is optimal. However, for writing, the lamp should be positioned on the side of the nondominant hand to avoid shadows (Figueiro, 2001). When addressing lighting, it is important to consider glare and its potential negative influence on performance. Glare can be managed through use of filters, window sheers, no-wax polish, and lamp shades.

Four Level I studies (Bowers et al., 2001; Brunnström et al., 2004; Eldred, 1992; Eperjesi et al., 2007) and two Level II studies (Fosse & Valberg, 2004; Haymes & Lee, 2006) in the systematic review focused on the effectiveness of illumination as a means of improving older adults' ability to read and improve leisure and social participation. Although the studies provided moderate

evidence to support the influence of illumination on reading speed (Bowers et al., 2001; Eldred, 1992), no evidence supported a particular type of light source, such as fluorescent, incandescent, or halogen (Brunnström et al., 2004; Eperjesi et al., 2007; Haymes & Lee, 2006).

In general, older adults with low vision typically require illumination levels of 1,000 to 7,000 lux (typical room lighting is 500–600 lux, and home lighting is typically 50 lux) to optimally perform reading activities (Bowers et al., 2001; Eldred, 1992), even though they often prefer lower-than-optimal illumination levels. Therefore, because each client's vision is unique, optimal illumination levels should be determined individually for each client (Eldred, 1992; Fosse & Valberg, 2004).

Contrast Strategies and Summary of the Evidence to Support Contrast Strategies

Normative aging changes such as opacification of the human lens and ocular disease create a decreased ability to detect or a decreased sensitivity to color and contrast (Figueiro, 2001). The inability to differentiate subtle variations in color or distinguish an object from its background can impair the older adult's ability to complete ADLs. Being able to distinguish the road from the curb may be difficult with reduced contrast sensitivity; however, when that same curb is highlighted by red or yellow markings, it is easier to navigate and safety is improved. Likewise, drinking coffee from a white cup rather than a black cup may make identifying the amount of coffee in the cup easier. Increasing the contrast between the object and its background is a simple way of increasing its visibility. Improving lighting and contrast in the environment can assist with independence and safety, because impaired contrast has been linked to increased risk of falls (Lord, 2006).

The systematic review found minimal evidence to support or refute the effectiveness of contrast as a general intervention strategy for older adults with low vision. However, Eperjesi, Fowler, and Evans (2004) examined the effects of 10 colored light-filter overlays on the reading rate of people with AMD in a Level I study. They found no significant relationship between the colors of the filters and reading rate. Overall, they found no evidence supporting the use of a colored overlay to improve reading requirements for the performance of daily occupations by older adults with low vision. Use of contrast strategies, such as yellow marking tape, colored filters, or using a white plate on a black placemat, can improve a client's participation in desired occupations (Eperjesi et al., 2004). In a Level II, nonrandomized control study, Wolffsohn, Dinardo, and Vingrys (2002) found a subjective benefit of the use of yellow filters for adults with AMD, with a slight enhancement in contrast sensitivity. Eperjesi and colleagues (2004) found that CPF450 lenses (yellow/orange) improved reading speed by 5%–15% for participants with AMD.

Nonoptical Strategies

Nonoptical strategies such as bold-lined paper, typoscopes (writing guides), or large-print items often are used as interventions to maintain participation in desired occupations. If a person is having difficulty with writing tasks, some nonoptical strategies that can be helpful are bold-lined paper, bold-line pens (20/20 pen), or writing guides. These strategies increase writing legibility by orienting the person or improving the visibility of the space allowed.

When minimal magnification is required, or when optical devices are not a viable option, large print may be a successful intervention strategy. Many large-print items are commercially available or easy to make on your own, such as address books, leisure items (playing cards, bingo cards, crossword puzzles, or word searches), medication labels (by request at the pharmacy), health management devices (such as blood pressure cuffs or glucometers), household management items (e.g., thermostats, clocks), or books at the library or bookstore.

Summary of the Evidence to Support Nonoptical Strategies

The systematic review found minimal evidence to support or refute the effectiveness of nonoptical strategies for older adults with low vision. However, specific evidence was found with regard to text characteristics, a large-print reading home program, and the use of a line guide within an optical magnifier. Those results are presented here.

Russell-Minda and colleagues (2007) completed a systematic review of 18 research studies examining the legibility of various typefaces for people with low vision. They found inconclusive evidence regarding serifs, although they did find a subjective preference for sans serif typefaces such as Arial, Verdana, Helvetica, and Adsans over Times New Roman. They also found that no consensus exists on a standard font size for low vision printed materials. However, they recommended a font size of at least 16 to 18 points, boldface, on white paper for maximized readability and legibility. They also concluded that adequate spacing between letters provides an advantage to people with low vision.

In a study that provided Level II evidence, Cheong and colleagues (2005) researched whether using large-print reading material at home with and without a reduced field of view, in addition to brief in-office practice, improves reading performance. The results provided no support for the use of a large-print reading home program before learning how to use an optical magnifier because no significant difference was found in reading rates among the three groups. However, this study was not adequately powered because the sample size was not large enough to yield generalizable findings.

In a Level III study, Cheong, Bowers, and Lovie-Kitchin (2009) examined the effects of using a line guide with a stand magnifier on the reading performance of older adults with AMD. They found that use of a line guide resulted in a small decrease in reading speed. Despite this finding, 48% of participants actually preferred using it, reporting that it provided better orientation than reading with a stand magnifier without a line guide. The nature of this study's design did not provide the quality evidence needed to support or refute the effectiveness of using a line guide with an optical magnifier during reading tasks. Therefore, more research is needed in this area.

Driving and Community Mobility

Often, vision loss results in a person having to retire from driving. However, vision loss also can increase one's risk of falls (Lord & Dayhew, 2001) and have an impact on one's ability to ambulate or navigate safely within the environment and community (Womack, 2012). Driving cessation and mobility impairment have been linked to decreased independence and quality of life (Hassell, Lamoureux, & Keeffe, 2006), increased rates of depression (Whittle & Goldenberg, 1996), decreased social and leisure participation (Desrosiers et al., 2009), and decreased balance and strength (Skelton, 2001).

Older adults with minimal to moderate low vision may still meet the minimum standards for restricted driver's licenses or bioptic driving in some states. In these cases, driving rehabilitation typically is recommended for comprehensive training, assessment, and modifications to the automobile, as necessary. The reader is referred to AOTA's *Occupational Therapy Practice Guidelines for Driving and Community Mobility for Older Adults* (Stav, Hunt, & Arbesman, 2006) for best practice in driving rehabilitation. (For license requirements by state, refer to www.nhtsa.gov/people/injury/olddrive/modeldriver/3_app_b.htm.)

People who do not meet these requirements must explore alternate transportation and community mobility. Most larger cities have some form of public transit, such as buses or subways, that run on set schedules to designated locations. Someone with low vision may find it difficult to identify a bus number or read the schedule of pickups. Physical access issues to use of these types of services also may exist, such as inability to manage the low-contrast stairs or escalators in dark subway stations.

Paratransit also may be available to an older adult with low vision. This type of transportation is usually done as an appointment or scheduled pick-up and is typically a curb-to-curb service. If an older adult cannot manage the steps in the home or locate the doctor's office in a large office building, however, paratransit still may present difficulties. In addition, because of scheduling, people often spend many hours waiting for their rides because other people may need to be picked up and dropped off. However, arm-in-arm or door-to-door services may be available in some areas. Many private transportation options also are available, ranging from organized volunteers at local senior centers to hired rides.

Community mobility often is impaired by visual acuity, visual field defects, or both; deficits in contrast sensitivity, color vision, or depth perception; environmental factors such as lighting and glare; and other age-related and systemic issues. Maintaining mobility and participation in desired activities is important for general health and well-being. The occupational therapy practitioner working with an older adult with low vision should be able to teach the client and his or her family sighted-guide techniques (refer to Table 4). These techniques allow the client a sense of control and comfort while being guided in the environment. Additional techniques include trailing, protective stance, teaching or encouraging self-advocacy, or being able to request or accept assistance when needed. The occupational therapy practitioner also can refer the client to an orientation and mobility specialist for training in the use of a long cane and to provide more specific training in orientation to space in relation to the physical environment.

The occupational therapy practitioner can assist the client in learning systematic scanning techniques to help orient him or her to the environment (refer to the "Visual Skills Training" section). This systematic scanning can alert the client to hazards in his or her environment before ambulation. The occupational therapy practitioner also can train the client in the use of optical devices as prescribed

Table 4. Strategies to Promote Community Mobility for Older Adults With Low Vision

Sighted-Guide Technique

1. Introduce yourself and ask the person whether he or she would like assistance.
2. The person with visual impairment should be positioned to your side and slightly behind you.
3. The person with visual impairment should grasp your elbow (by placing the back of his or her hand against yours, the person can travel up your arm to your elbow). The person's arm should be positioned at 90° and held close to his or her body.
4. Walk at a normal, slightly slower gait.
5. You are responsible for keeping the person safe, so it is important to verbalize hazards or obstacles that are in the environment, for example, doors or steps.
6. In narrow areas, such as doorways, you can slip your arm behind the person's back and have him or her get behind you to navigate the narrow walkway. Once through, you can reposition your arm to get back into the beginning position. (Gense & Gense, 2004)

Trailing

1. Position yourself about 6 in. from a wall; extend your arm out a foot in front of you at hip level with the palm of your hand against the wall.
2. Walk forward using the palm of your hand to identify any objects in your way.

Protective Stance

Upper body: Arm is held out at shoulder height, with elbow bent and parallel to the floor, palm facing forward; protects from objects at head or chest level.

Lower body: Arm is extended down and diagonal across the body with palm outward; protects trunk and legs.

---

by the low vision optometrist or ophthalmologist. Prisms, mirrors, and reverse telescopes all have been used to improve awareness of the visual field.

Prisms are used to shift an image from the nonseeing area into the seeing area. For field awareness, Fresnel prisms typically are used. These temporary press-on prisms are placed on the person's glasses, with the base of the prism placed toward the visual field defect.

Similarly, mirrors can be used to improve awareness of the visual field defect. Mirrors can be attached to a client's glasses and, using scanning, the client can look into the mirror to see areas that are outside his or her visual field.

Last, a reverse telescope can be used. Looking through the telescope in reverse minifies the image rather than magnifying it, providing a greater visual field. However, as the image is minified, it also becomes less clear, so reverse telescopes are used only in low powers. The person must not walk while looking through the telescope; it is used for spotting only. The occupational therapist must also understand the role of an orientation

mobility specialist (see Table 5) and refer the client to the specialist for additional training when necessary.

Summary of the Evidence to Support Driving and Community Mobility

The evidence on the effectiveness of occupational therapy interventions for driving and community mobility for older adults with visual impairment is limited. The strongest evidence has supported patient education and driving rehabilitation programs, with noted improvements in self-regulatory behavior and improved quality-of-life measures (Lamoureux et al., 2007 [Level III]; Owsley, McGwin, Phillips, McNeal, & Stalvey, 2004 [Level I]; Stalvey & Owsley, 2003 [Level II]). In addition, training in the use of bioptics also has been found beneficial for improvements in simulated and on-road driving skills and outdoor mobility skills (Bowers, Peli, Elgin, McGwin, & Owsley, 2005 [Level III]; Laderman, Szlyk, Kelsch, & Seiple, 2000 [Level III]; Szlyk et al., 1998 [Level II], 2000 [Level III], 2005 [Level I]).

Problem Solving and Self-Management

The use of active problem-solving strategies in a group or individual setting may be a useful strategy to facilitate engagement in occupations of choice, improve self-management skills, improve self-efficacy, and reduce symptoms of depression. Facilitating problem solving with older adults with vision loss can promote participation in ADLs, IADLs, and leisure and social activities (Brody et al., 1999; Dahlin Ivanoff et al., 2002; Eklund & Dahlin-Ivanoff, 2007; Girdler, Boldy, Dhaliwal, Crowley, & Packer, 2010; Rovner & Casten, 2008).

For older adults with vision loss, the ability to problem solve may be compromised by their level of adjustment to or acceptance of their visual impairment; for example, a person who is still in search of a cure for his or her ocular disease may not be ready to identify compensatory strategies. Problem solving requires insight into the deficits or challenges faced; an unclear or poor understanding of the impact of vision loss on occupational performance or the permanence of the vision loss can significantly limit rehabilitation potential.

Occupational therapy practitioners have the skills to teach their clients problem-solving strategies for self-management whereby problems are defined, realistic goals are established, solutions are generated and implemented, and outcomes are evaluated (Rovner & Casten, 2008). For example, an older adult may want to continue volunteering at the local children's hospital, which would include setting smaller goals such as independently arranging transportation or reading large-print books to the children. The occupational therapy practitioner and the client continue to work together to determine solutions and strategies to meet the goals, such as using a large-print, high-contrast, preprogrammed telephone; an illuminated handheld magnifier; filters to decrease glare and increase contrast; or books on tape or compact disc. After the potential solutions are determined and the client has received training in using them, the most appropriate strategy is implemented. Last, the outcome of the strategy is evaluated, in this case, evaluating whether the client is able to participate in his or her volunteer work.

Summary of the Evidence to Support Problem Solving and Self-management

Strong evidence has supported the use of problem-solving strategies to increase participation in ADLs, IADLs, and leisure and social participation and to improve self-management skills. For ADL and IADL performance, the systematic review included three Level I studies (Brody et al., 1999; Eklund & Dahlin-Ivanoff, 2007; Girdler et al., 2010) and one Level II study (Birk et al., 2004), which found significant improvements in either the Activity Card Sort or a self-report questionnaire on daily tasks. For leisure and social participation, the systematic review included three Level I studies, which found that problem solving is related to increased participation in leisure and social participation among older adults with AMD (Brody et al., 1999; Dahlin Ivanoff et al., 2002; Rovner & Casten, 2008).

Brody and colleagues (1999) found that group problem-solving training with support of peers or professionals improved engagement in leisure and social participation. With participation in health education and problem-solving groups, older adults gained a sense of security, confidence, and control in leisure and social participation as well as in ADL performance (Dahlin Ivanoff et al., 2002; Rovner & Casten, 2008).

Eklund and Dahlin-Ivanoff (2007) found that with individual and group health promotion programs, people had improved use of low vision optical and nonoptical devices. Brody and colleagues (1999) compared a self-management group intervention with no treatment. The group consisted of six 2-hour sessions involving educational presentations and problem-solving practice. Participants increased their use of LVDs and reported an increase in some activities, such as gardening, and continued performance in other activities, such as walking. However, participants also reported a decline in other occupations, such as attending religious events.

Similarly, Dahlin-Ivanoff and colleagues (2002) found that a group problem-solving approach including eight 2-hour weekly sessions led by an occupational therapist resulted in improvements in perceived security in daily occupations, with the most significant improvements found in reading an article, writing a note, and reading a billing statement. Rovner and Casten (2008) compared a problem-solving training program with usual care. The training focused on assisting the participants in defining the problem; establishing realistic goals; generating, choosing, and implementing possible solutions; and then evaluating the outcomes. Participants who received the problem-solving training were more likely to continue with valued occupations. Likewise, Girdler and colleagues (2010) compared usual care with a self-management group intervention and found that participants who received the self-management intervention were more likely to continue to participate in valued activities and experienced an improvement in health outcomes.

Advocacy

Many services and potential intervention strategies frequently used in working with older adults with low vision often are not covered by third-party payers. For example, optical and electronic LVDs are not traditionally reimbursable expenses. As a result, occupational therapy practitioners often advocate for their clients to obtain the needed devices, modifications, or referral services to maximize occupational performance. Writing grants or obtaining used equipment for clients is often necessary to allow clients to obtain the necessary devices.

Supporting the client in self-advocating for the necessary services or modifications to support independence and safety is also important. For instance, a client who lives in public housing can request modifications to his or her apartment under reasonable accommodations. Providing the client with the necessary knowledge of community resources can assist him or her in self-advocacy and maximize independence in valued occupations.

Multidisciplinary and Multicomponent Interventions

The occupational therapy practitioner often works on a multidisciplinary team that may include ophthalmologists, opticians, orientation and mobility specialists, low vision therapists, lighting experts, social workers, psychologists, and others (refer to Table 5 to understand the roles of the various team members). Occupational therapy practitioners must understand the role of each member of the multidisciplinary team and refer clients when appropriate to ensure optimal outcomes.

Refer to the case illustration in Box 4.

In addition to a multidisciplinary approach to low vision rehabilitation, the systematic review

---

Box 4. Case Study: Additional Low Vision Rehabilitation Team Members

Ophthalmologist: **Lillian** consistently sees her retina specialist every 6 months to monitor her retinal health. Currently, Lillian's macular degeneration is stable.

Low vision optometrist: Lillian recently saw her low vision specialist, who referred her to occupational therapy for services. Lillian returns to the Low Vision Clinic when changes in her vision interfere with her desired occupations.

Orientation and mobility specialist: Lillian was referred to the orientation and mobility specialist to explore community mobility and use of public transportation systems.

Table 5. Low Vision Practitioners

Type of Practitioner	Role on the Low Vision Team
Ophthalmologist	Physician who specializes in diagnosis and management of eye disease. Some specialize in vision rehabilitation or work with clients with eye disease and refer them for vision rehabilitation services. Responsible for the medical management of the eye, medical or surgical.
Optometrist	Eye care practitioner responsible for nonsurgical management of the eye. Treatments include lenses, medications, vision therapy, and low vision rehabilitation. Responsible for the prescription of low vision devices.
Orientation and mobility specialist	Provides training for clients with low vision or blindness regarding orientation in space in relation to the physical environment; training in the use of long cane; and training in home and community mobility, including the use of public transportation.
Vision rehabilitation therapist	Teaches techniques, technology, and use of devices for people with low vision or blindness. Emphasizes effect of visual impairment on activities of daily living, patient, and family.
Teacher for children with visual impairment	Provides specialized training to children who have visual impairment or blindness. Teaches techniques, Braille, technology, and use of devices for people with low vision or blindness.
Rehabilitation counselor	Provides counseling related to occupation and employment, provides career guidance, and assists with job placement (from teaching interviewing skills to adjusting to the workplace).
Certified low vision therapist	Teaches patients to use their vision more efficiently, with and without optical devices; environmental modification; and visual skills training.

Sources. Kern and Miller (1997); Scheiman, Scheiman, and Whittaker (2007); Sokol-McKay and Michels (2005); Studebaker and Pankow (2004).

found strong evidence for the use of multicomponent patient education and training. The occupational therapy practitioner often combines the intervention strategies described earlier to create a multicomponent intervention plan that is optimal for each client. For example, a client with AMD would like to be independent in meal preparation. Interventions that may facilitate independence may include developing visual skills such as eccentric viewing or scanning strategies; training in the use of optical or electronic magnification devices to read instructions or recipes; training in the use of nonoptical strategies, such as large-print recipes; using sensory and visual substitution strategies, such as bump dots to mark the stove or a say-when device to ensure safety when pouring; maximizing organizational strategies, such as alphabetizing spices; modifying the environment, such as improving the lighting in the meal preparation area; training in safe mobility strategies; learning active problem solving; and advocating for needed services, such as food delivery.

Refer to the case illustration in Box 5 for occupational therapy interventions.

Summary of the Evidence to Support Multidisciplinary Low Vision Rehabilitation Programs That Include Occupational Therapy

The systematic review found strong evidence supporting low vision rehabilitation programs that included occupational therapy as part of the services offered (Eklund & Dahlin-Ivanoff, 2007; Eklund, Sjöstrand, & Dahlin-Ivanoff, 2008; Markowitz, Kent, Schuchard, & Fletcher, 2008; McCabe, Nason, Demers Turco, Friedman, & Seddon, 2000; Pankow, Luchins, Studebaker, & Chettleburgh, 2004). Four articles provide Level I evidence (Eklund & Dahlin-Ivanoff, 2007; Eklund et al., 2008; McCabe et al., 2000; Pankow et al., 2004), and one article provides Level III evidence (Markowitz et al., 2008). The services that were carried out by occupational therapists included a combination of the following:

Box 5. Case Study: Occupational Therapy Intervention

After educating **Lillian** on her ocular condition and identifying her goals, the therapist initiated intervention. On the basis of current evidence, the therapist used a multicomponent approach to her plan of care.

Lillian's goals were as follows:
- Independence in money management
- Independence in medication management
- Independence in meal preparation and cooking for herself and her family
- Independence in reading for leisure.

Learning active problem solving:

Current evidence supports the use of problem-solving strategies to improve everyday activities and leisure and social participation. Because Lillian has age-related macular degeneration and is likely to have changes in her vision and visual function, active problem-solving strategies were used throughout her intervention. Helping Lillian to identify the problem, generate strategies to implement, and assess the outcomes will assist her in remaining independent in desired activities today and help her in adjusting to future vision changes.

Training in the use of optical or electronic magnification devices:

The evidence for the use of optical or electronic magnification devices to improve reading speed and decrease disability for older adults with low vision is moderate to weak. Multiple devices were trialed with Lillian to determine best fit. For short spotting tasks, a 3.5× light-emitting diode handheld magnifier was determined to allow Lillian to read her medication labels and recipes. Because of decreased contrast, a stand magnifier was difficult for Lillian to use for extended reading. With the help of her local Lion's Club, Lillian was able to obtain a closed-circuit television (CCTV) for extended reading tasks. Training in proper use of devices was provided. After training, Lillian was able to return to previous reading tasks, reading mail, medications, labels, and short stories for leisure (although she was able to read with efficiency, she became fatigued in extended reading tasks).

Visual skills:

Even though the evidence for visual skills training for older adults with low vision is weak, the therapist used this intervention strategy as part of the multicomponent approach to Lillian's care. Lillian was aware of her central scotoma, and her preferred retinal locus (PRL) was identified to be at a 2 o'clock position. Eccentric viewing training focused on improving awareness of the central scotoma and improved use of her new PRL. Training began with static tasks, learning to move the scotoma out of the way to observe an object, then advancing to more complex tasks. She learned to use the steady eye technique with her CCTV, in which she was able to maintain her eccentric position and moved the text by eye vs. scanning across the page to read.

(Continued)

Box 5. Case Study: Occupational Therapy Intervention *(Cont.)*

Modifying the environment:
Lillian's home had several hazards. Her family was instructed to remove all throw rugs. Because of reduced contrast, Lillian had difficulty identifying the depth and rise of stairs; high-contrast tape was used to mark the edge of all steps. She was recommended to position a gooseneck table lamp over her right shoulder and onto the task when working at her kitchen table (reading and writing tasks). Under-cabinet lighting was recommended in her food preparation area. A large-print calendar and 20/20 pen were recommended for maintaining her appointment schedule. These modifications to the environment are supported by moderate to weak evidence.

Using visual substitution strategies (tactile and auditory):
Lillian struggled to see dials on appliances. After high-contrast orange bump dots were used to mark settings on the stove, microwave, washer, and dryer, Lillian was able to set the appliances independently. Because of fatigue with extended reading, Lillian was provided with books on tape, which allowed her to continue with her book group and her primary leisure pursuit. These substitution strategies are supported by weak evidence.

Maximizing organizational strategies:
Despite insufficient evidence, organizational strategies were used as part of the multicomponent intervention approach to Lillian's care. Because Lillian struggled at times with finding items in the home, the occupational therapist instructed Lillian to (1) consistently place items in their home location; (2) keep items orderly and keep phone numbers and addresses in order; (3) pair like items, such as socks, shoes, or outfits; and (4) develop a routine for cleaning. The therapist also worked with Lillian's family to make sure they were consistent with organization.

Training in appropriate community mobility strategies:
Lillian no longer drives and uses family and friends for transportation. Her family was educated in sighted-guide techniques.

Advocating for needed services:
Because low vision devices were not covered by her insurance companies, a grant request was written on Lillian's behalf to her local Lion's Club to obtain a CCTV.

- Group therapy (Eklund & Dahlin-Ivanoff, 2007; Eklund et al., 2008)
- Educating clients about their condition and providing additional information and resources (Eklund & Dahlin-Ivanoff, 2007; Eklund et al., 2008)
- Training in problem-solving strategies (Eklund & Dahlin-Ivanoff, 2007; Eklund et al., 2008)
- Environmental modifications (McCabe et al., 2000)
- Training in the use of LVDs (Markowitz et al., 2008; McCabe et al., 2000; Pankow et al., 2004)
- Instruction in adaptive techniques, energy conservation, and work simplification (McCabe et al., 2000)

- Training in proper reading techniques (Markowitz et al., 2008)
- Training in daily activities and occupational themes (e.g., self-care, communication, orientation and mobility, food preparation, shopping, financial management, cleaning; Eklund & Dahlin-Ivanoff, 2007; Eklund et al., 2008).

Other health professionals participating in the programs include ophthalmologists, optometrists, nurses, social workers, psychologists, opticians, low vision therapists, and lighting experts.

Specifically, McCabe and colleagues (2000) compared an individual low vision program including optometry, occupational therapy, and social work with one that also included a family member in all intervention sessions. They concluded that although they found no difference between the two intervention groups, clients in both groups demonstrated significant gains in visual capacity and decreased dependence in daily activities such as reading newspapers, sewing, and visiting friends. Likewise, Pankow and colleagues (2004) found a significant difference in the ability to perform daily occupations, including social and leisure participation, between those who participated in a low vision program and those who did not. This program began with collaborative goal setting followed by any of the following relevant services: provision of optical aids, blind rehabilitation teaching, orientation and mobility training, driving rehabilitation, and occupational therapy. Markowitz and colleagues (2008) performed a nonrandomized one-group study and concluded that a low vision rehabilitation program specifically improves the ability of older adults with low vision to read medication labels.

Eklund and Dahlin-Ivanoff (2007) and Eklund and colleagues (2008) compared an occupational therapy–based health promotion group program with individual intervention. The group program also involved low vision professionals including an ophthalmologist, optician, low vision therapist, and a lighting professional, whereas the individual-

ized program did not. The researchers concluded that those receiving the health promotion program were less dependent in performing ADLs (Eklund & Dahlin-Ivanoff, 2007). Participants in the health promotion program used a combination of LVDs and ADL devices, whereas participants in the individualized program primarily used LVDs (Eklund & Dahlin-Ivanoff, 2007). Over a 28-month period, those in the health promotion program were able to maintain their ability to perform daily occupations (Eklund et al., 2008).

The low vision programs described in these articles are somewhat diverse in that each suggests a different model of providing low vision rehabilitation services. However, in combination, these studies provide strong evidence that low vision programs including occupational therapy services and other low vision professionals improve the ability of older adults with low vision to perform the reading necessary for participation in daily occupations. They also provide moderate evidence that a combination of low vision services improves leisure and social participation among older adults with low vision.

Summary of the Evidence to Support Multidisciplinary Low Vision Rehabilitation Programs That Did Not Include Occupational Therapy

We should note that the systematic review included five additional original research articles reporting on the effectiveness of low vision programs in improving reading for the performance of occupations (Goodrich, Kirby, Wood, & Peters, 2006; La Grow, 2004; Reeves, Harper, & Russell, 2004; Scanlan & Cuddeford, 2004; Stelmack et al., 2008). However, unlike the articles discussed in the preceding section, these programs did not include occupational therapy as part of their comprehensive services. Therefore, the findings from these articles were considered separately from those of articles that specifically included occupational therapy services. These comprehensive programs typically consisted of a combination of services that included a low vision examination, diagnosis and prognosis of the eye condition, education regarding the condition, low vision therapy, prescription of an LVD, eccentric viewing, home visits, or all of these.

Of these five studies, three provided Level I evidence through randomized controlled trials (Reeves et al., 2004; Scanlan & Cuddeford, 2004; Stelmack et al., 2008), one provided Level II evidence (La Grow, 2004), and one provided Level III evidence (Goodrich et al., 2006). The studies found conflicting evidence regarding the effectiveness of low vision rehabilitation programs on improving reading performance (and activities that involved reading) when compared with an alternate intervention (Goodrich et al., 2006; La Grow, 2004; Reeves et al., 2004; Scanlan & Cuddeford, 2004). Moreover, the evidence to support the effectiveness of these programs over receiving no intervention is limited (Stelmack et al., 2008).

Another four studies in the systematic review, which provided moderate evidence, discussed multidisciplinary programs that did not include occupational therapy–specific services that addressed leisure and social participation among older adults with low vision. One provided Level II evidence (La Grow, 2004), and three provided Level III evidence (Elliott & Kuyk, 1994; Hinds et al., 2003; Shuttleworth, Dunlop, Collins, & James, 1995). In summary, each of these studies evaluated integrated low vision programs that included services provided by a variety of practitioners, including but not limited to ophthalmologists, optometrists, ophthalmic nurses, social workers, and blindness rehabilitation professionals, and found that they resulted in improved engagement in leisure activities and social participation. Many of the intervention strategies used in these interdisciplinary low vision services would be within the scope of occupational therapy practice.

Summary of the Evidence to Support Multicomponent Client Education and Training

Three Level I trials (Brody et al., 2002; Eklund & Dahlin-Ivanoff, 2007; Girdler et al., 2010) and one

Level II trial (Birk et al., 2004) in this systemic review provide evidence to support the use of multicomponent patient education and training for older adults with low vision. Each of these trials used a well-defined patient education program to teach patients how to cope with various issues of low vision.

These multicomponent programs used, respectively, multiple sessions of a self-management program (Brody et al., 2002; Girdler et al., 2010), a health promotion program (Eklund & Dahlin-Ivanoff, 2007), or a psychosocial intervention program (Birk et al., 2004). The intervention content included low vision education, optical device training, problem-solving skills training, information and resources sharing, and homework assignments and discussions.

On completion of the program, all intervention groups showed significant improvement in either the Activity Card Sort or self-report questionnaires on daily tasks. The retention of treatment effect at follow-up is uncertain. Two trials showed that the effect could last for 1 month (Girdler et al., 2010) or even 1 year after the program (Eklund & Dahlin-Ivanoff, 2007), but one trial showed a long-term benefit at 6 months only for participants with depression (Brody et al., 2002).

In summary, strong evidence supports a multidisciplinary approach to low vision rehabilitation, including occupational therapy and occupational therapy programs that use multiple intervention strategies (Birk et al., 2004; Brody et al., 2002; Eklund & Dahlin-Ivanoff, 2007; Girdler et al., 2010). Although no one clearly defined model of low vision rehabilitation or one combination of intervention strategies is most successful, occupational therapy services that include multiple intervention strategies combined with other low vision professional interventions may be most beneficial to older adults with low vision.

Intervention Review

Intervention review is a continuous process of reevaluating and reviewing the intervention plan, the effectiveness of its delivery, progress toward targeted outcomes, and the need for future occupational therapy and referrals to other agencies or professionals (AOTA, 2008). Reevaluation may involve readministering assessments used at the time of initial evaluation, a satisfaction questionnaire completed by the client, or questions that evaluate each goal (Berg, 1997; Minkel, 1996). Reevaluation normally substantiates progress toward goal attainment, indicates any change in functional status, and directs modification of the intervention plan, if necessary (Moyers & Dale, 2007).

Outcome Monitoring

Occupational therapists and occupational therapy assistants document outcomes in discharge evaluations or discontinuation notes (AOTA, 2013). This documentation should be completed "within the time frames, formats, and standards established by practice settings, agencies, external accreditation programs, and payers" (AOTA, 2010, p. 417). A focus on outcomes is interwoven throughout the process of occupational therapy (AOTA, 2008), and occupational therapists should contribute their patient data and perspective to comprehensive team-based outcome assessments.

The COPM is a common outcome assessment measure that can be used with older adults with low vision (Law et al., 1990). If used during initial evaluation to determine the client's specific goals for the rehabilitation process, it can be readministered as needed during and at the conclusion of rehabilitation to determine progress made toward those goals. Law and colleagues (2004) stated that a change of at least 2 points from the original assessment scores on the 10-point performance and satisfaction scales indicates a clinically significant change.

On the basis of the client's stated goals, other outcome measurement tools may be used to gather additional outcome data on specific changes in occupational performance. For example, the Melbourne Low-Vision ADL Index (MLVAI; Haymes et al., 2001) or the Impact of Vision Impairment (IVI;

Lamoureux et al., 2004) may be readministered to determine changes in ADL or IADL performance. Informal assessment of occupational performance, such as direct observation, also may be useful in outcome monitoring. Although informal assessment is by definition not standardized and therefore cannot be used for broader purposes such as programmatic assessment, it does allow for a qualitative description of the change in performance of a meaningful activity.

Occupational therapists working with older adults with low vision often focus on outcomes emphasizing an adaptation to or compensation for performance skills such as reading and writing. Specifically, readministering assessments of reading and writing is a useful way to gain objective information about changes in an older adult's ability to perform these skills in a timely, accurate, or legible manner. Often, these assessments can be used with or without an LVD (either optical or electronic magnification), so changes in performance resulting from visual skills training or appropriate device use can be captured as needed at the time of reassessment. The MNRead Acuity Charts (Mansfield et al., 1994), the Visual Skills for Reading (the Pepper Test; Watson et al., 1995), and the Low Vision Reading Comprehension Assessment (Watson, Wright, & Long, 1996) are three potentially useful outcome measurement tools in the area of reading performance. Likewise, the Low Vision Writing Assessment (Watson, Wright, et al., 2004) can be used to reassess writing performance.

Environmental modifications made during the low vision rehabilitation process also can be monitored and recorded. For example, a light meter can be used to quantify lighting levels in each of the commonly used areas of the home environment before making modifications to task lighting and ambient lighting levels. All key areas throughout the home should be included in this monitoring. Moreover, photographs may be a useful way to document outcomes in environmental modifications that are often a part of the low vision rehabilitation intervention plan such as changes in contrast in the bathroom and kitchen areas.

In addition to monitoring outcomes of older adults with low vision, occupational therapists use aggregate data from outcome assessments to evaluate the effectiveness of specific interventions and programs. Working together with other members of the low vision rehabilitation team, collection of standardized outcomes data contributes to program development and the establishment of a research foundation for evidence-based practice.

Refer to the case illustration in Box 6 for outcome measures and discharge status.

Discontinuation, Discharge Planning, and Follow-Up

The existing U.S. health care reimbursement system bases eligibility for medical rehabilitation, length of stay, and discharge from services on physical impairment, including visual impairment, that interferes with occupational performance. Occupational therapists' strength in analyzing and adapting daily activities can be of great assistance in helping older adults with low vision resume meaningful roles and occupations.

Because of the progressive nature of age-related eye disease, clients may require occupational therapy services intermittently throughout the course of the disease process. For example, training in higher powered optical devices, use of eccentric viewing techniques, or sensory substitution strategies that were not indicated earlier may be needed in later stages of the disease process. In addition, normative aging changes, comorbidities, and chronic disease may have an impact on the course of rehabilitation or require additional services or referrals.

Discharge planning should begin during the evaluation process with consideration of the needs and desires of the client and his or her significant others. Discontinuation of services should occur when (1) the client achieves his or her established goals, (2) a plateau in progress is reached, (3) the client is unable or no longer wants to participate in the rehabilitative process, or (4) skilled occupational therapy services are no longer needed. Considerations for discharge also should include referrals to community services (such as support groups) or specialized services (such as orientation and mobility specialists) and ongoing follow-up on eye care services and potential need for skilled occupational therapy services as the condition or client needs change.

Occupational Therapy Services for Organizations and Populations

Occupational therapists may work with organizations such as businesses, industries, or agencies that serve older adults with low vision in a variety of ways by

- Providing consultation or educational information to community groups;
- Developing programs or grant proposals for funding agencies to develop community programs for older adults with low vision;
- Serving on the advisory boards of visual impairment support groups to establish services and programs for older adults with low vision and their families;
- Consulting for community groups of older adults with low vision who are engaging in self-advocacy efforts to fund LVDs and adapt environments to meet their capabilities and needs;
- Consulting on job tasks and environmental structures for local businesses who employ older adults with low vision; and
- Consulting for the state department of health to evaluate existing occupational therapy services for older adults with low vision and recommend or assist in developing improved methods, services, and programs.

Occupational therapists who provide services to organizations that serve individuals including older adults with low vision enter the therapeutic relationship with respect for the values and beliefs of the organization. They seek to understand the collective abilities and needs of the organization's members and how the features and structure of the organization support or inhibit the overall performance of people in the organization (AOTA, 2008). The

Box 6. Case Study: Outcome Measures and Discharge Status

Canadian Occupational Performance Measure (COPM) Results

Performance Area	Importance	Performance	Satisfaction
Self-care Personal care: Medication management	10	9	8
Self-care Community management: Finances	7	9	8
Productivity Household management: Cooking	9	9	9
Leisure Quiet recreation: Reading	9	8	8

COPM Performance Score 1: 35/4 = 8.75
COPM Satisfaction Score 1: 25/4 = 8.25

Activity of daily living (ADL) status: Lillian is independent in all ADL and instrumental ADL tasks using low vision devices and compensatory strategies.

Eccentric Viewing and Preferred Retinal Locus (PRL): Lillian is aware of her central scotoma and is able to use her PRL for distance and near tasks.

Collins Low Vision Writing Assessment:

Writing grocery list	10/10
Writing/recording checks	10/10
Written language	10/10
Reading notes to self	9/10
Completing a form	10/10
Total score:	49/50

Pepper Visual Skills Test:
Accuracy score: 95%
Words/minute: 100
Errors: Misidentification

Lillian's goals:
• Independence in money management (goal met)
• Independence in medication management (goal met)
• Independence in meal preparation and cooking for herself and her family (goal met)
• Independence in reading for leisure (goal met).

skills of an occupational therapist with experience in community-based programming, program development, and management and reimbursement can assist community organizations and agencies in dealing with the issues and needs of older adults with low vision. Therapists work to affect the organization's design and ability to more effectively and efficiently meet the needs of older adults with low vision and other stakeholders while empowering members with low vision to seek satisfying lives.

Occupational therapists may facilitate occupational justice for older adults with low vision by assisting groups of people with low vision to organize to address social policies, actions, and laws that enable people to engage in meaningful occupations and ensuring that older adults with low vision are considered in ongoing discussions on health care reform. They may lobby for legislation that funds community programming, prevention education, or access to appropriate housing. Occupational therapists may volunteer in community advocacy and prevention activities that enhance the health of all people by engaging in activities such as educating community groups on prevention activities to minimize the incidence of low vision; creating a donation system for LVDs; fundraising or grant writing to support environmental adaptations; advocating for accessible outdoor spaces; or lobbying state legislature for funding prevention and educational programming.

Implications of the Evidence for Occupational Therapy Research

Although the systematic reviews of occupational therapy for older adults with low vision revealed that the amount of evidence available to support occupational therapy intervention for this client population is increasing, the need to enhance the current literature with further research continues. The research supported several intervention strategies, but in some cases the small participant population,

lack of control groups, or decreased total number of research studies supporting a particular intervention strategy made the overall strength of evidence limited. Certainly, further research is needed to support occupational therapy for older adults with low vision, including research with larger sample sizes and with a variety of low vision diagnoses.

One area of research that deserves further study is the composition of the low vision rehabilitation team and the development of model low vision rehabilitation programs. The systematic reviews revealed several research studies evaluating the effectiveness of an overall low vision program. However, these programs lacked consistency in which low vision professionals were on the team, their roles, the number of therapy sessions the older adult with low vision received, and types of interventions that were included in the program (Eklund & Dahlin-Ivanoff, 2007; Eklund et al., 2008; Goodrich et al., 2006; La Grow, 2004; Markowitz et al., 2008; McCabe et al., 2000; Pankow et al., 2004; Reeves et al., 2004; Scanlan & Cuddeford, 2004; Stelmack et al., 2008), which made it difficult to evaluate them consistently. Although the overall finding indicated that multidisciplinary teams that include occupational therapy are effective (Eklund & Dahlin-Ivanoff, 2007; Eklund et al., 2008; Markowitz et al., 2008; McCabe et al., 2000; Pankow et al., 2004), further research to clarify the most effective overall program and team composition is needed.

In addition to research that examines occupational therapy intervention within the context of the multidisciplinary team, additional research is needed to further examine specific occupational therapy intervention strategies. For example, the results of the systematic review indicate that moderate evidence supports the use of stand-based electronic magnification to increase the reading speed of older adults with low vision. However, a growing number of new electronic magnification options continue to be commercially available to older adults with low vision. The rapid advancements in technology will demand increased research on the effectiveness of these new devices.

Other areas in need of further research include visual skills training, organizational strategies, and community mobility. The systematic review found limited evidence for these intervention strategies. Therefore, increasing the number of high-quality studies to evaluate these specific strategies would assist with evidence-based treatment planning and potentially lead to improved outcomes for this client population.

Finally, future research also must incorporate the promotion of functional health literacy or the ability to gather, interpret, and use information to make suitable health-related decisions (AOTA, 2011), not only for the general population but also for the older adult population. Functional health literacy must be considered, especially when providing services to older adults with visual impairment to maximize their understanding and incorporation of occupational therapy practitioners' skilled recommendations into their daily lives.

Additionally, because low vision in the older adult population is often comorbid with depression, cognitive decline, hearing loss, and physical limitations from a variety of conditions (Perlmutter et al., 2010), future research needs to consider how people with multiple health limitations can successfully manage their health and continue to participate in meaningful occupations. It is crucial that future research address these considerations, because research remains the gateway to the ongoing delivery of progressive interventions and services to people with low vision. More specific recommendations based on the findings from the systematic reviews on older adults with low vision are found in Table 6.

Implications of the Evidence for Occupational Therapy Education

Although low vision can present as a single diagnosis, it is more frequently combined with other comorbidities, chronic diseases, and general age-related functional decline such as stroke, diabetes mellitus, arthritis, and dementia. Therefore, older adults with low vision often face multiple functional impairments addressed in the course of an occupational therapist's academic preparation, which can lead to a potentially overwhelming number of impairments in a single client and can challenge a student's ability to prioritize treatment goals and select intervention approaches. Occupational therapy curricula must contain comprehensive information on the visual system as well as on neurological, sensorimotor, psychosocial, and cognitive components of human function to prepare students to meet the needs of the older adult with low vision in a holistic manner.

Educators presenting information on older adults with low vision need to simultaneously present existing evidence supporting occupational therapy interventions and integrate literature published by optometrists, ophthalmologists, low vision professionals, and other members of the low vision multidisciplinary team into lectures and lesson plans. Exposing students to existing and newly developed standardized assessments for use with the low vision population is required not only by accreditation standards but also by ethical obligations to adequately prepare the next generation of occupational therapy practitioners. Students must learn to systematically examine the effect of their interventions and develop the habit of applying their research competencies in everyday practice to support or negate particular interventions with clients (Holm, 2000). Students and practicing occupational therapists must examine their intervention by observing closely; interpreting observations; reflecting on goals, outcomes, and intervening variables; and experimenting with therapy variations to determine the key therapeutic processes.

In addition to a strong grounding in evidence to support intervention strategies and standardized assessment tools, educators also must be current in the assistive technologies that are used with older adults with low vision. Students should be trained in the correct use of magnification devices, both electronic and optical, so that they are prepared

Table 6. Recommendations for Occupational Therapy Interventions for Older Adults With Low Vision

Recommended	No Recommendation	Not Recommended
Use of problem-solving strategies to increase participation in ADL and IADL tasks and leisure and social participation (A)	Colored overlays do not improve reading performance (B)	
Multicomponent patient education and training to improve occupational performance (A)	Preferential use of either binocular or monocular viewing for reading performance (I)	
Increased illumination to improve reading performance (B)	Use of a specific light source (I)	
Increased illumination to improve social participation (B)		
Stand-based magnification systems to increase reading speed and duration (B)		
Patient education programs to improve self-regulation in driving and community mobility (B)		
Use of bioptics to improve simulated and on-road driving skills as well as outdoor mobility skill (B)		
Contrast and typeface (sans serif), type size (14–16 points), and even spacing to improve legibility and readability of print (B)		
Use of contrast, for example, yellow marking tape, colored filters, using a white plate on a black placemat, to improve participation in occupations (C)		
Use of low-vision devices (e.g., high-add spectacles, nonilluminated and illuminated hand-held magnifiers, nonilluminated and illuminated stand magnifiers, high plus lenses, telescopes, electronic magnifiers [such as closed-circuit TVs]) to improve reading speed and reduce level of disability when performing ADL tasks (C)		
Eccentric viewing training to improve reading performance (C)		
Eccentric viewing in combination with instruction in magnification to improve reading (C)		
Eccentric viewing completed with specific software programs for near vision and ADLs (C)		
Use of optical magnifiers versus head-mounted magnification systems to improve reading speed (C)		
Use of sensory substitution strategies (e.g., talking books) to maintain engagement in desired occupations (C)		
Use of contrast to improve reading performance: colored overlays (I)		
Use of spectacle reading glasses to improve reading performance (I)		
Use of organizational strategies to compensate for vision loss (I)		

Note. Criteria for level of evidence (A, B, C, I, D) are based on standard language (Agency for Healthcare Research and Quality, 2009). Suggested recommendations are based on the available evidence and content experts' clinical expertise regarding the value of using the intervention in practice. ADL = activities of daily living; IADL = instrumental activities of daily living; A = strong evidence that occupational therapy pracftitioners should routinely provide the intervention to eligible clients; good evidence that the intervention improves important outcomes and concluded that benefits substantially outweigh harm; B = moderate evidence that occupational therapy practitioners should routinely provide the intervention to eligible clients; at least fair evidence that the intervention improves important outcomes and concluded that benefits outweigh harm; C = weak evidence that the intervention can improve outcomes, and the balance of the benefits and harms may result either in a recommendation that occupational therapy practitioners routinely provide the intervention to eligible clients or in no recommendation because the balance of the benefits and harm is too close to justify a general recommendation; I = insufficient evidence to determine whether occupational therapy practitioners should be routinely providing the intervention; evidence that the intervention is effective is lacking, of poor quality, or conflicting and the balance of benefits and harm cannot be determined; D = recommend that occupational therapy practitioners do not provide the intervention to eligible clients; at least fair evidence that the intervention is ineffective or that harm outweighs benefits.

to train their clients in the use of these devices in the clinical setting. Knowledge about appropriate lighting strategies, visual skills training, sensory substitution strategies, contrast techniques, problem-solving skills, and general awareness of the range of assistive devices available for the older adult with low vision beyond magnification should be considered essential features of occupational therapy education in the area of low vision.

Because low vision is a common secondary diagnosis in the older adult population, intervention can occur across traditional settings of fieldwork ranging from outpatient clinics to long-term care. Students need to recognize that a secondary diagnosis of low vision can influence the outcome of intervention, and addressing low vision is therefore critical to the success of the overall therapy program even when it is not the primary diagnosis. Additionally, exposing students to community-based practice settings in which older adults with low vision receive services can assist them not only in learning to think outside the medical model but also addressing client-centered goals to "support health and participation in life through engagement in occupation" (AOTA, 2008, p. 626).

Continued efforts to bridge the gap between research and practice can be achieved by increasing research partnerships between faculty and students from academic programs and occupational therapists in clinical settings providing services to older adults with low vision. These research partnerships can lead to meaningful evidence supporting occupational therapy practice with the low vision population.

Implications of the Evidence for Occupational Therapy Clinical Practice

The literature has provided an abundance of information about the negative effects of vision loss on ADLs and IADLs, reading, community mobility, and leisure and social participation among older adults. However, the evidence supporting the effectiveness of occupational therapy interventions to address these needs is somewhat limited. Occupational therapy interventions to facilitate engagement in occupation that have moderate to strong research evidence support include problem-solving training; training in the use of LVDs, especially electronic magnification devices; and proper illumination. In addition, when provided as part of a multidisciplinary team approach to low vision rehabilitation and when using a multicomponent education program for maintaining performance of ADLs and IADLs, occupational therapy intervention also has been shown to be effective. Although the evidence is limited, instruction in optical magnifiers and visual skills training also may be considered.

Some commonly used occupational therapy intervention strategies such as sensory substitution, large print, contrast, organizational strategies, and community mobility have limited support from quantitative data. Qualitative studies have shown the impact of vision loss on older adults' occupational performance. The use of these compensatory and adaptive strategies have been found to be essential for maintaining quality of life and adjusting to vision loss (Girdler, Packer, & Boldy, 2008; Stevens-Ratchford & Krause, 2004). However, additional intervention studies are needed that specifically look at the outcomes of occupational therapy interventions for older adults with low vision.

The use of active problem-solving strategies in group and individual settings may be helpful in maintaining engagement in occupations of choice, improved self-efficacy, and reduction of depressive symptoms. Occupational therapy practitioners must be able to teach their clients problem-solving skills, including defining the problem, establishing realistic and measurable goals, developing and implementing solutions, and evaluating the outcomes (Brody et al., 1999; Dahlin Ivanoff et al., 2002; Rovner & Casten, 2008).

Strong evidence supports the use of electronic magnification, and limited evidence supports the use of optical magnification specifically for reading tasks (Bowers et al., 2001; Cheong et al., 2005;

Culham et al., 2004; Goodrich & Kirby, 2001; Goodrich et al., 2004; Horowitz et al., 2006; Margrain, 2000; Nguyen et al., 2009; Peterson et al., 2003; Stelmack et al., 1991). To ensure proper use and care, training in use of these LVDs is essential. It is also important that clients understand the progressive nature of their ocular condition and the potential need for future optical devices. In addition, clients should understand that not all devices will work for every activity, and they may need several LVDs to engage in a variety of occupations.

It is crucial that practitioners consider these results while keeping in mind that every client with low vision has unique preferences in terms of the various components of low vision rehabilitation. For example, one must consider that stand-based electronic systems are not ideal for some reading activities, and not all older adults have the financial capacity to obtain electronic magnification systems. Therefore, prescribed optical devices may be a suitable alternative to electronic magnification in some cases (Peterson et al., 2003; Stelmack et al., 1991). Occupational therapy practitioners must take into account the needs of each client in terms of the reading tasks the client wants to perform, the natural environment in which he or she performs these tasks, and the client's financial situation. By applying a holistic approach in practice, practitioners can remain client-centered and ultimately determine the most appropriate interventions to meet each client's unique needs.

Occupational therapy practitioners also must address their clients' lighting needs. Although the evidence does not support any one type of lighting (Eperjesi et al., 2007; Haymes & Lee, 2006), moderate evidence supports the use of illumination as an effective intervention strategy for the performance of reading tasks (Bowers et al., 2001; Eldred, 1992). The average older adult requires 3–4 times greater illumination than a younger person. Older adults with low vision may require even greater levels of illumination (Figueiro, 2001; Sanford, 1997). However, lighting is often complicated by issues such as source of light, glare, contrast, and balance of lighting levels.

Effective lighting must be tailored to the individual and the specific task because different visual conditions may require different solutions. General considerations for lighting should include increased lighting levels, glare control, increased contrast, balanced or uniform lighting levels, and enhanced color perception and color rendering (Figueiro, 2001; Noell-Waggoner, 2004). Figueiro (2001) and the Illuminating Engineering Society of North America (2007) have made some recommendations for lighting levels for older adults to help support productive aging, including ambient lighting of 300 lux and task-specific lighting of 1,000 lux.

A multicomponent education program is the most effective intervention to maintain or improve ADL and IADL performance (Birk et al., 2004; Brody et al., 2002; Eklund & Dahlin-Ivanoff, 2007; Girdler et al., 2010). The multicomponent education program provides older adults with the knowledge to address issues that they may face in their own homes. The programs often last several weeks, allowing for older adults to learn new skills and apply them in their own contexts. The programs are usually in a group format, which also serves as peer support. In addition, use of a multidisciplinary team approach—which could include optometrists, occupational therapy practitioners, orientation and mobility specialists, social workers, and psychologists or provision of multiple services by a single practitioner—has been found to be beneficial (Eklund & Dahlin-Ivanoff, 2007; Eklund et al., 2008; Markowitz et al., 2008; McCabe et al., 2000; Pankow et al., 2004). The type and duration of interventions should be client-centered and tailored to the client's needs.

Lastly, occupational therapy practitioners working with older adults with vision loss must address alternative transportation systems available in the community. Most older adults with low vision will retire from driving or restrict their driving (Womack, 2012), which can restrict their access to desired occupations. Exploration of available transportation in the community can help maintain leisure and social participation, assist with IADL completion, and improve quality of life (Womack, 2012).

Appendix A. Preparation and Qualifications of Occupational Therapists and Occupational Therapy Assistants

Who Are Occupational Therapists?

To practice as an occupational therapist, the individual trained in the United States

- Has graduated from an occupational therapy program accredited by the Accreditation Council for Occupational Therapy Education (ACOTE®) or predecessor organizations;
- Has successfully completed a period of supervised fieldwork experience required by the recognized educational institution where the applicant met the academic requirements of an educational program for occupational therapists that is accredited by ACOTE or predecessor organizations;
- Has passed a nationally recognized entry-level examination for occupational therapists; and
- Fulfills state requirements for licensure, certification, or registration.

Educational Programs for the Occupational Therapist

These include the following:

- Biological, physical, social, and behavioral sciences

- Basic tenets of occupational therapy
- Occupational therapy theoretical perspectives
- Screening evaluation
- Formulation and implementation of an intervention plan
- Context of service delivery
- Management of occupational therapy services (master's level)
- Leadership and management (doctoral level)
- Professional ethics, values, and responsibilities.

The fieldwork component of the program is designed to develop competent, entry-level, generalist occupational therapists by providing experience with a variety of clients across the lifespan and in a variety of settings. Fieldwork is integral to the program's curriculum design and includes an in-depth experience in delivering occupational therapy services to clients, focusing on the application of purposeful and meaningful occupation and/or research, administration, and management of occupational therapy services. The fieldwork experience is designed to promote clinical reasoning and reflective practice, to transmit the values and beliefs that enable ethical practice, and to develop professionalism and competence in career responsibilities. Doctoral-level students also must complete a doctoral experiential component designed to develop advanced skills beyond a generalist level.

Who Are Occupational Therapy Assistants?

To practice as an occupational therapy assistant, the individual trained in the United States
- Has graduated from an occupational therapy assistant program accredited by ACOTE or predecessor organizations;
- Has successfully completed a period of supervised fieldwork experience required by the recognized educational institution where the applicant met the academic requirements of an educational program for occupational therapy assistants that is accredited by ACOTE or predecessor organizations;
- Has passed a nationally recognized entry-level examination for occupational therapy assistants; and
- Fulfills state requirements for licensure, certification, or registration.

Educational Programs for the Occupational Therapy Assistant

These include the following:
- Biological, physical, social, and behavioral sciences
- Basic tenets of occupational therapy

- Screening and assessment
- Intervention and implementation
- Context of service delivery
- Assistance in management of occupational therapy services
- Professional ethics, values, and responsibilities.

The fieldwork component of the program is designed to develop competent, entry-level, generalist occupational therapy assistants by providing experience with a variety of clients across the lifespan and in a variety of settings. Fieldwork is integral to the program's curriculum design and includes an in-depth experience in delivering occupational therapy services to clients, focusing on the application of purposeful and meaningful occupation. The fieldwork experience is designed to promote clinical reasoning appropriate to the occupational therapy assistant role, to transmit the values and beliefs that enable ethical practice, and to develop professionalism and competence in career responsibilities.

Regulation of Occupational Therapy Practice

All occupational therapists and occupational therapy assistants must practice under federal and state law. Currently, 50 states, the District of Columbia, Puerto Rico, and Guam have enacted laws regulating the practice of occupational therapy.

Note. The majority of this information is taken from the *2011 Accreditation Council for Occupational Therapy Education (ACOTE) Standards* (ACOTE, 2012).

Appendix B.
Selected *Current Procedural Terminology*™ *(CPT)* Codes for Occupational Therapy Evaluations and Interventions for Older Adults With Low Vision

The following chart can guide occupational therapists in making clinically appropriate decisions in selecting the most relevant *CPT* code to describe occupational therapy evaluation and intervention for older adults. Occupational therapy practitioners should use the most appropriate code from the current *CPT* manual on the basis of specific services provided, individual patient goals, payer coding and billing policy, and common usage.

Examples of Occupational Therapy Evaluation and Intervention	Suggested *CPT* Codes
Evaluation	
Consists of the initial evaluation of the older adult's status and performance in areas of occupation, performance skills, performance patterns, context and environment, activity demands, and client factors. • Perform functional evaluation using standardized assessments (e.g., Canadian Occupational Performance Manual, Brain Injury Visual Assessment Battery for Adults). • Use nonstandardized assessment methods, such as observation of the client performing tasks that require visual function such as reading mail, managing medications, cooking, or applying make-up.	**97003**—Occupational therapy evaluation

(Continued)

Examples of Occupational Therapy Evaluation and Intervention	Suggested *CPT* Codes
• Gather data from various other sources (e.g., medical record, occupational profile, interview, caregivers, significant others). • Develop individual goals to address performance deficits or enhance strengths.	
Formal reassessment of changes in performance resulting from changes in status or diagnosis or if intervention plans need significant revisions. • Reassessment of an older adult's status and progress, usually after a change in patient status, using standardized and non-standardized assessments.	97004—Occupational therapy reevaluation
• Administer, interpret, and report findings from assistive technology assessment to identify technology to improve an older adult's specific area of function, such as the use of a portable magnification system.	97755—Assistive technology assessment (e.g., to restore, augment, or compensate for existing function, optimize functional tasks, or maximize environmental accessibility), direct one-on-one contact by provider, with written report, each 15 minutes
• Participate in a medical team conference as part of a diagnostic or evaluation team whereby the team discusses the evaluation findings, diagnoses, and recommendations with a client and his or her family.	99366—Medical team conference with interdisciplinary team of health care professionals, face-to-face with patient or family, 30 minutes or more, participation by nonphysician qualified health care professional
• Participate in a medical team conference as part of a diagnostic or evaluation team whereby the team reviews evaluation findings and clarifies diagnostic considerations and recommendations before meeting with a client and his or her family.	99368—Medical team conference with interdisciplinary team of health care professionals, patient or family not present, 30 minutes or more, participation by nonphysician qualified health care professional
Intervention	
Intervene through modulation (facilitation and inhibition) of sensory input and stimulation of motor responses using neuromuscular reeducation and neurorehabilitation approaches. • Application of neurorehabilitation techniques to facilitate motor and sensory processing and promote adaptive responses to sitting, standing, and posturing to facilitate participation in desired occupation (e.g., using a computer, playing catch with grandchildren). • Develop and train in use of motor responses to effect change in functional performance and limit risk of fall (e.g., toileting, toilet transfers, bathing, tub transfers).	97112—Therapeutic procedure, one or more areas, each 15 minutes; neuromuscular reeducation of movement, balance, coordination, kinesthetic sense, posture, or proprioception for sitting or standing activities
• Use of selected individualized therapeutic activities as an intervention to improve performance of specific functional tasks (e.g., use of a light training board to improve visual scanning or therapeutic activities to increase hand dexterity or coordination to use low-vision devices).	97530—Therapeutic activities, direct (one-on-one) patient contact by the provider (use of dynamic activities to improve functional performance), each 15 minutes

(Continued)

Examples of Occupational Therapy Evaluation and Intervention	Suggested *CPT* Codes
• Develop compensatory methods (e.g., medication timer or planner) to provide auditory cueing to take medication. • Develop and instruct older adult in compensatory strategies for completion of daily home management activities such as meal preparation and clothes washing. • Train in methods of adapting bathroom, bathing routine, and habits to improve safety and independence for bathing task.	**97535**—Self-care and home management training (e.g., activities of daily living) and compensatory training, meal preparation, safety procedures, and instruction in use of assistive technology devices and adaptive equipment, direct one-on-one contact by provider, each 15 minutes
• Provide individualized intervention focusing on community or work integration. • Teach community mobility skills using public or alternative transportation methods. • Instruct an older adult in driving retraining skills to help compensate for visual impairment after a stroke.	**97537**—Community or work reintegration training (e.g., shopping, transportation, money management, avocational activities, and work environment or modification analysis, work task analysis, use of assistive technology device or adaptive equipment), direct one-on-one contact by provider, each 15 minutes
• Direct group activities for two or more clients to support a common goal, such as learning problem-solving strategies or organizational strategies. • Provide group intervention focusing on diabetic self-management techniques that include low vision–related techniques.	**97150**—Therapeutic procedure or procedures, group (two or more individuals; group therapy procedures involve constant attendance by the physician or therapist but by definition do not require one-on-one patient contact by the physician or therapist)

Note. Medical team conferences are not billable to Medicare; however, these codes may be useful for reporting productivity. These codes do not represent all of the possible codes that may be used in occupational therapy evaluation and intervention. Not all payers will reimburse for all codes. Codes shown refer to *CPT 2013*. Refer to *CPT 2013* for the complete list of available codes.

CPT codes are updated annually. New and revised codes become effective January 1. Always refer to the updated annual *CPT* publication for most current codes.

CPT 2013™ is a trademark of the American Medical Association. *Current Procedural Terminology (CPT)* five-digit codes, two-digit codes, modifiers, and descriptions are copyright © by the American Medical Association. All rights reserved.

Appendix C.
Evidence-Based Practice

Occupational therapists and occupational therapy assistants, as do many other health care professionals facing the demands of payers, regulators, and consumers, increasingly have to demonstrate clinical effectiveness. In addition, they are eager to provide services that are client-centered, supported by evidence, and delivered in an efficient and cost-effective manner. Over the past 20 years, evidence-based practice (EBP) has been advocated widely as one approach to effective health care delivery.

Since 1998, the American Occupational Therapy Association (AOTA) has instituted a series of EBP projects to assist members with meeting the challenge of finding and reviewing the literature to identify evidence and, in turn, using this evidence to inform practice (Lieberman & Scheer, 2002). Following the evidence-based philosophy of Sackett, Rosenberg, Muir Gray, Haynes, and Richardson (1996), AOTA's projects are based on the principle that the EBP of occupational therapy relies on the integration of information from three sources: (1) clinical experience and reasoning, (2) preferences of clients and their families, and (3) findings from the best available research.

A major focus of AOTA's EBP projects is an ongoing program of systematic reviews of the multidisciplinary scientific literature, using focused questions and standardized procedures to identify practice-relevant evidence and discuss its implications for practice, education, and research. Systematic reviews of literature relevant to low vision in older adults strengthen understanding of the foundations of this important area of practice.

According to Law and Baum (1998), *evidence-based occupational therapy practice* "uses research evidence together with clinical knowledge and reasoning to make decisions about interventions that are effective for a specific client" (p. 131). An evidence-based perspective is founded on the assumption that scientific evidence of the effectiveness of occupational therapy intervention can be judged to be more or less strong and valid according to a hierarchy of research designs, an assessment of the quality of the research, or both. AOTA uses standards of evidence modeled on those developed in evidence-based medicine.

This model standardizes and ranks the value of scientific evidence for biomedical practice using the grading system presented in Table C.1. In this system, the highest level of evidence, *Level I*, includes systematic reviews of the literature, meta-analyses, and randomized controlled trials (RCTs). In RCTs, participants are randomly allocated to either an intervention or a control group, and the outcomes of both groups are compared. In *Level II* studies, assignment to a treatment or a control group is not randomized (cohort study); *Level III* studies do not have a control group; *Level IV* studies use a single-case experimental design, sometimes reported over several participants; and *Level V* studies use case reports and expert opinion that include narrative literature reviews and consensus statements.

These systematic reviews were initiated and supported by AOTA as part of the Evidence-Based Practice project. In 2009, both the AOTA National Office and members expressed interest in developing an EBP guideline on occupational therapy for older adults with low vision because of the increased incidence of older adults with low vision and AOTA's interest in focusing on areas related to

Table C.1. Levels of Evidence for Occupational Therapy Outcomes Research

Evidence Level	Definition
I	Systematic reviews, meta-analyses, randomized controlled trials
II	Two groups, nonrandomized studies (e.g., cohort, case control)
III	One group, nonrandomized (e.g., before and after, pretest and posttest)
IV	Descriptive studies that include analysis of outcomes (e.g., single-subject design, case series)
V	Case reports and expert opinion that include narrative literature reviews and consensus statements

Note. From "Evidence-Based Medicine: What It Is and What It Isn't," by D. L. Sackett, W. M. Rosenberg, J. A. Muir Gray, R. B. Haynes, & W. S. Richardson, 1996, *British Medical Journal, 312*, pp. 71–72. Copyright © 1996 by the British Medical Association. Adapted with permission.

board and specialty certification. It was felt that the EBP guideline would provide occupational therapy practitioners with findings that would guide and support practice in this area. In addition, a practice guideline would be used to support the role of occupational therapy with external audiences. Four focused questions were developed for the systematic reviews of occupational therapy interventions for older adults with low vision. The questions were generated in conjunction with an advisory group of content experts in low vision within and outside of occupational therapy.

The following focused questions from the review are included in this Practice Guideline:

1. What is the evidence for the effectiveness of environmental interventions within the scope of occupational therapy practice to maintain, restore, and improve performance in activities of daily living (ADLs) and instrumental activities of daily living (IADLs) within the home for older adults with low vision?

2. What is the evidence for the effectiveness of providing interventions within the scope of occupational therapy practice to improve the ability to use optical, nonoptical, and electronic magnifying devices to complete the reading required for performance of occupations by older adults with low vision?

3. What is the evidence for the effectiveness of interventions within the scope of occupational therapy practice to improve the driving performance and community mobility of older adults with low vision?

4. What is the evidence for the effectiveness of interventions within the scope of occupational therapy practice to maintain, restore, and improve performance in leisure and social participation for older adults with low vision?

Method

Search terms for the reviews were developed by the consultant to the AOTA Evidence-Based Practice Project and AOTA staff in consultation with the authors of each question and reviewed by the advisory group. The search terms were developed not only to capture pertinent articles but also to make sure that the terms relevant to the specific thesaurus of each database were included. Table C.2. lists the search terms related to populations and interventions included in each systematic review. A medical research librarian with experience in completing systematic review searches conducted all searches and confirmed and improved the search strategies.

Inclusion and exclusion criteria are critical to the systematic review process because they provide the structure for the quality, type, and years of publication of the literature incorporated into a review. The review for all four questions was limited to peer-reviewed scientific literature published in English. It also included consolidated information sources such as the Cochrane Collaboration.

Table C.2. Search Terms for Systematic Reviews on Older Adults With Low Vision

Category	Key Search Terms
Population	Aging, elderly, older adults, seniors plus age-related macular degeneration, cataracts, central visual impairment, diabetic retinopathy, glaucoma, hemianopsia, low vision, macula, neurological impairment, partial vision, peripheral visual impairment, retina, retinitis pigmentosa, Stargardt's disease, visual disorders, visual fields, visual impairment, visually impaired persons
Intervention—participation in activities of daily living and instrumental activities of daily living	Activities of daily living (bathing, dressing, eating, toileting, walking), instrumental activities of daily living (cooking, shopping, medication management, telephone, money management), acoustic/audio cues, adaptive equipment, adaptive techniques, aging in place, ambient lighting, appliance marking, assistive technology, color, compensation, contrast, contrast sensitivity, dark–light adaptation, depression, eccentric, environment, environmental intervention, environmental modification/adaptation, fall prevention, falls, glare, glare control, illuminance, illumination, intervention, labeling, large print, life space, lighting, low vision rehabilitation, marking, mobility, occupational therapy, organization, pattern, quality of life, reading speed or rate, rehabilitation, safety, scotoma awareness, spectral filters, tactile cues, tactile marking, task lighting, trip hazards, vision training, visual cues, visual environment
Intervention—reading with magnifying and other devices	Activities of daily living, adaptive equipment, aging in place, assistive technology, audio device, bifocals, bioptics, client education, closed-circuit television (CCTV), contrast/contrast sensitivity, depression, device training, eccentric viewing, electronic magnification, electronic reading software/device, ergonomics, instrumental activities of daily living, large print, low vision aid, low vision rehabilitation, low vision training, magnification, medication label, microscopes along with glasses, microscopic glasses, MNRead Acuity Chart, nonoptical device, occupational therapy, optical device, optics, Pepper Visual Skills for Reading Test, portable electronic magnifiers, preferred retinal locus, prescription label, prisms, quality of life, reading and writing (menu reading, newspaper reading, recipe reading), reading comprehension, reading device, reading fluency, reading rate, reading speed, relative distance, relative size, scotoma awareness, sensory aids, spectacles, telescopes, video magnification, Web design
Intervention—driving and community mobility	AARP/Car Fit, bioptic driving, bioptic lens, bioptics, community mobility, community integration, contrast/contrast sensitivity, depression, driver training, driving, driving evaluation, field enhancement, field expansion, glare, intervention, low vision rehabilitation, prisms, processing speed, program effectiveness, quality of life, reaction time, restrictive licensing, traffic safety, transportation, transportation options for older adults, useful field of view, vision training, visual fields
Intervention—leisure and social participation	Accessibility, activity limitation, activity performance, adaptation, adaptive equipment, adjustment, adjustment to vision loss, assistive technology, community mobility, compensation, compensatory techniques, coping, cultural activities, daily living, depression, engagement/loneliness, environmental modification, environments, family, gardening, illumination, intervention, leisure (including specific leisure such as television watching, reading, travel, mobile phone use, mobility, access to transportation), leisure activity, leisure time physical activity, life satisfaction, longitudinal, mental health, occupational therapy, participation, passive leisure time, physical activity, problem solving, psychosocial adaptation, quality of life, recreation, recreational activity, rehabilitation, resources, scotoma awareness, socialization, social participation, social pursuits, social support, sports, stress, task lighting, vision-related quality of life, volunteer, well-being

The literature included in the review was published from 1990 to 2010, and the study populations were older adults, primarily ages 65 years or older, with low vision. Studies included in the review were of intervention approaches within occupational therapy's domain and scope of practice. The review excluded data from presentations, conference proceedings, non–peer-reviewed research literature, dissertations, and theses. Only Level I, II, III evidence was included in the reviews.

A total of 2,356 citations and abstracts were reviewed. The search related to ADL and IADL participation resulted in 510 references; the optics question, 268; the driving question, 973; and the leisure and social participation question, 605. The consultant to the EBP project completed the first step of eliminating references on the basis of citation and abstract. The reviews were carried out as academic partnerships in which academic faculty worked with occupational therapy graduate students to carry out the reviews. Review teams completed the next step of eliminating references on the basis of further review of citations and abstracts. The full-text versions of potential articles were retrieved, and the review teams determined final inclusion in the review on the basis of predetermined inclusion and exclusion criteria.

A total of 70 articles were included in the final review. Table C.3. presents the number and level of evidence for articles included in each review question. The teams working on each focused question reviewed the articles according to their quality (scientific rigor and lack of bias) and level of evidence. Each article included in the review then was abstracted using an evidence table that provides a summary of the methods and findings of the article and an appraisal of the strengths and weaknesses of the study on the basis of design and methodology.

The strength of the evidence is based on the guidelines of the U.S. Preventive Services Task Force (http://www.uspreventiveservicestaskforce. org/uspstf/grades.htm). The designation of *strong evidence* includes consistent results from well-conducted studies, usually at least two RCTS. A designation of *moderate evidence* may be made on the basis of one RCT or two or more studies with lower levels of evidence. In addition, some inconsistency of findings across individual studies might preclude a classification of strong evidence. The designation of *limited evidence* may be based on few studies, flaws in the available studies, and some inconsistency in the findings across individual studies. A designation of *mixed* may indicate that the findings were inconsistent across studies in a given category. A designation of *insufficient* evidence may indicate that the number and quality of studies is too limited to make any clear classification.

Review authors also completed a Critically Appraised Topic (CAT), a summary and appraisal of the key findings, clinical bottom line, and implications for occupational therapy based on the articles included in the review for each question.

Table C.3. Number of Articles in Each Review at Each Level of Evidence

Review	Evidence Level					
	I	II	III	IV	V	Total
Participation in activities of daily living and instrumental activities of daily living	9	5	3	0	0	17
Reading with magnifying and other devices	16	8	8	0	0	32
Driving and community mobility	4	2	2	0	0	8
Leisure and social participation	9	1	3	0	0	13
Total	38	16	16	0	0	70

AOTA staff and the EBP project consultant reviewed the evidence tables and CATs to ensure quality control.

Strengths and Limitations of the Systematic Reviews

The systematic reviews presented in this Practice Guideline cover many aspects of occupational therapy practice for older adults with low vision and have several strengths. Four focused questions were included in the reviews, covering information related to several aspects of the domain of occupational therapy addressed in the *Occupational Therapy Practice Framework* (2nd ed.; AOTA, 2008). The reviews included 70 articles, and three-fourths of the articles were Level I and II evidence.

The reviews involved systematic methodologies and incorporated quality control measures. Please refer to the individual systematic reviews (Berger, McAteer, Schreier, & Kaldenberg, 2013; Justiss, 2013; Liu, Brost, Horton, Kenyon, & Mears, 2013; Smallfield, Schaefer, & Myers, 2013) for complete information on the results and their implications.

Limitations of the studies incorporated in the reviews may include small sample size and lack of long-term follow-up. Depending on the level of evidence, the studies may lack randomization and a control group. In addition, separating out the effects of a single intervention that is part of a multimodal intervention is difficult. Also, many of the studies used outcome measures not specifically geared to the systematic review question, which may have obscured the ability to separate out the effect of the interventions studied on the targeted outcome.

Appendix D.
Evidence Tables

Table D.1. Summary of Evidence on Interventions to Improve Performance of Daily Activities at Home for Older Adults With Low Vision

Author/Year[a]	Study Objectives	Level/Design/Participants[b]	Intervention and Outcome Measures	Results	Study Limitations
Birk et al. (2004)	To evaluate the effectiveness of a group psychosocial intervention program	Level II—Quasi-experimental design. *Participants* $N = 22$ participants with AMD and visual acuity < 20/70 Intervention group $n = 14$ Comparison group $n = 8$ Mean age = 73 yr	*Intervention* The intervention group received 6 modules of psychosocial intervention (muscle relaxation, problem solving, exchange of experience and information) delivered at the study site by 2 clinical psychologists in 5 group sessions over 5 wk. Intervention with the comparison group was not reported. *Outcome Measure* Modified MAI: ADL and IADL ability at posttest (5 wk).	The intervention group had higher ADL and IADL ability as measured by the MAI compared with the comparison group.	Sample size was small. Group sizes were unequal (14 vs. 8). No attention control group was used.
http://dx.doi.org/10.1093/geront/44.6.836					
Brody et al. (2002, 2005)	To assess the effectiveness of a self-management program	Level I—Randomized control trial. *Participants* $N = 231$ patients with advanced AMD and visual acuity < 20/60 Intervention group $n = 86$ Attention control group $n = 73$ Control group $n = 72$	*Intervention* The intervention group received a 6-wk, 12-hr self-management program led by a health professional in a community conference room. The program included didactic presentations and group problem solving with guided practice. The attention control group received a tape-recorded health education program with health lectures. The control participants were on a wait list. *Outcome Measure* NEI VFQ–25: Low vision–specific quality of life at postintervention and 6 mo.	The intervention group showed significant improvement in functioning at posttest. At 6 mo, only those who were depressed in the intervention group showed improvement.	No limitations were noted.
http://dx.doi.org/10.1001/archopht.123.1.46	Mean age = 81 yr				

Study	Objective	Design/Level	Intervention and Outcome Measure	Results	Limitations
Brunnström et al. (2004)	To examine the effect of lighting on activities of daily living	Level III—One-group, pretest–posttest design. *Participants* N = 46 participants with impaired visual function (55% with macular disease) and visual acuity < 6/18 Mean age = 76 yr	*Intervention* A low vision therapist and a lighting expert provided basic lighting adjustment in the kitchen, hall, and bathroom. *Outcome Measure* Self-reported task performance at 6 mo.	Significant improvement was found in 2 kitchen tasks: pouring a drink and slicing bread. Performance of tasks in the hall deteriorated.	No data on reliability, validity, and responsiveness were reported for the outcome assessment. The researchers did not adjust for confounding factors in the analysis (e.g., magnitude of lighting change, progress of eye condition). No control group was used. Not every participant had lighting in all 3 areas adjusted.

http://dx.doi.org/10.1111/j.1475-1313.2004.00192.x

Study	Objective	Design/Level	Intervention and Outcome Measure	Results	Limitations
de Boer et al. (2006)	To compare the effects of two types of low vision service programs: optometric vs. multidisciplinary	Level II—Quasi-experimental design. *Participants* N = 215 participants with visual impairment (many with AMD) and visual acuity < 20/50 Optometric services group n = 116 Multidisciplinary services group n = 99 Mean age = 78 yr	*Intervention* The optometric services group received low vision services, including low vision aids and instructions, from an optometrist. The multidisciplinary services group received low vision services, including low vision aids and the services of occupational therapists, social workers, and psychologists, from a multidisciplinary rehabilitation center. *Outcome Measure* LVQOL: Reading and Fine Work subscale 12 mo after first visit.	Both groups had nonsignificant results in change scores between baseline and 1 yr.	The deterioration of vision was confounded with the outcome. The dropout rate was moderate (27%). The two groups were not matched.

(Continued)

Table D.1. Summary of Evidence on Interventions to Improve Performance of Daily Activities at Home for Older Adults With Low Vision (*Cont.*)

Author/Year[a]	Study Objectives	Level/Design/Participants[b]	Intervention and Outcome Measures	Results	Study Limitations
Eklund et al. (2004, 2008; Dahlin Ivanoff et al., 2002; Eklund & Dahlin-Ivanoff, 2007) http://dx.doi.org/10.1080/09638280400100162950 http://dx.doi.org/10.1080/1103812070144-2963 http://dx.doi.org/10.5014/ajot.56.3.322 http://dx.doi.org/10.1080/1748310070171471717	To determine the effectiveness of an activity-based health promotion program	Level I—Randomized control trial. *Participants* *N* = 131 patients with AMD and visual acuity < 0.1 Intervention group *n* = 62 Usual-care group *n* = 69 Mean age = 78 yr	*Intervention* The intervention group received usual care and an 8-wk health education program led by occupational therapists. Participants met in small groups once/wk for 2 hr at the clinic and discussed 8 different occupational themes. *Outcome Measures* • 28-item questionnaire: perceived security in performing daily activities at 4, 16, and 28 mo • ADL staircase test at 4, 16, and 28 mo.	The intervention group showed significant improvement in perceived security over time. The intervention group maintained the level of daily activities and showed slowdown in the disablement process.	The dropout rate was high (42%). The outcome assessor was not blinded to the intervention conditions.
Engel et al. (2000) http://dx.doi.org/10.1111/j.1600-0420.2004.00371.x	To examine the effectiveness of a local low vision rehabilitation service	Level III—One-group, pretest–posttest design. *Participants* *N* = 70 older adults with visual impairment Mean age = 76 yr	*Intervention* Service teachers provided an average of 7 hr of services in 5 home visits. *Outcome Measure* Scaled interview questionnaire.	No significant results were found for items related to ADLs.	The instrument's psychometric properties were poor. The content of services was not well defined.
Girdler et al. (2010; Packer et al., 2009)	To evaluate the effectiveness of a low vision self-management program	Level I—Randomized control trial. *Participants* *N* = 77 participants with age-related vision loss (most with AMD) and visual acuity ≤ 6/12 Intervention group *n* = 36 Usual-care group *n* = 41 Mean age = 79 yr	*Intervention* The intervention group received usual care plus an 8-wk self-management program in which participants met once a wk in groups of 6. An occupational therapist and a social worker delivered the program. *Outcome Measure* Activity card sort test at 8-wk posttest and 12 wk later.	The intervention group showed significant improvement at posttest and follow-up compared with the control group.	No limitations were noted.

Author/Year	Study Objectives	Level/Design/Participants	Intervention and Outcome Measures	Results	Study Limitations
La Grow (2004)	To compare the effects of two types of low vision service programs: comprehensive low vision service *vs.* noncomprehensive low vision service	Level II—Two groups matched on age, gender, and visual function. *Participants* *N* = 186 participants with visual impairment (50% mild) and visual acuity < 6/24 Comprehensive low vision group *n* = 93 Contrast group *n* = 93 Mean age = 81 yr	*Intervention* The comprehensive low vision group received a preclinical assessment, an initial low vision examination, training with any aids, and a follow-up home visit. The contrast group received assessment and instruction in independent living skills, orientation and mobility, and communications, as well as recreational and leisure activities. *Outcome Measures* • Adapted version of the Measure of Function and Psychosocial Outcomes of Blind Rehabilitation: IADLs at 6 mo and 12 mo • NEI VFQ–25 at 6 mo and 12 mo.	No significant differences were found between groups at posttest or follow-up.	The intervention was contaminated by services from a blindness foundation. The authors reported similarity between interventions provided to comprehensive and contrast groups.
Lamoureux et al. (2007) http://dx.doi.org/10.1167/iovs.06-0610	To evaluate the effectiveness of a multidisciplinary low vision rehabilitation program	Level III—One-group, pretest–posttest design. *Participants* *N* = 192 participants with visual acuity < 6/12; 62% had AMD and visual acuity < 20/40 Mean age = 80.3 yr	*Intervention* A multidisciplinary low vision rehabilitation team including occupational therapists provided the intervention; more than 2/3 of participants purchased low vision devices during the intervention. *Outcome Measures* • IVI Mobility and Independence subscale • Ability to read and access information at 3 to 6 mo.	No improvement, but approaching statistical significance (*p* = .07) in mobility and independence. Participants who received special services in orientation and mobility and also occupational therapy (*n* = 38) showed more gains on the Mobility and Independence subscale than those who did not. Significant improvement was found in reading and accessing information.	No control group was used. Participants did not use rehabilitation services equally (i.e., only some used occupational therapy services).

(Continued)

Author/Year[a]	Study Objectives	Level/Design/Participants[b]	Intervention and Outcome Measures	Results	Study Limitations
McCabe et al. (2000) http://dx.doi.org/10.1076/opep.7.4.259.4173	To test the effectiveness of involving family members in low vision rehabilitation	Level 1—Randomized control trial. *Participants* N = 97 participants with low vision (64% with AMD) and visual acuity < 20/100 Intervention (family-focused) group n = 49 Control group n = 48 Mean age = 69 yr	*Intervention* Both groups received multidisciplinary low vision rehabilitation that included occupational therapy. In the intervention group, family members were included in all rehabilitation sessions. In the control group, family members were excluded from all sessions. *Outcome Measures* • FAQ: ADLs and IADLs at posttest • FVPT: Ability to perform 4 visual tasks at posttest.	No difference was found between the treatment and control groups, although both improved in measured outcomes at posttest.	Family members' knowledge of low vision was not measured as an outcome.
Nilsson (1990)	To evaluate the effects of educational training in the use of optical aids and the use of residual vision	Level II—Quasi-experimental design. *Participants* N = 40 participants with AMD and visual acuity < 0.1 Intervention group n = 20 Comparison group n = 20 Mean age = 77 yr	*Intervention* The intervention group received visual aids from an ophthalmologist and training in the use of these aids from a low vision therapist. Of the group, 50% also had eccentric viewing training of about five 1-hr sessions. The comparison group received visual aids from an ophthalmologist and instructions on how to use them. *Outcome Measure* Ability to read newspaper headlines and text and TV titles and pictures at 1 mo.	A larger proportion of participants in the intervention group were able to read newspaper text and headlines and TV titles and pictures.	Outcome measures were not standardized tests.
Pankow et al. (2004)	To examine the effectiveness of a goal-attaining low vision rehabilitation program	Level 1—Randomized control trial. *Participants* N = 30 adults with low vision (majority with AMD) and visual acuity < 20/50 Intervention group n = 15 Control group n = 15 Mean age = 79 yr	*Intervention* The intervention group received vision rehabilitation, including occupational therapy, specifically geared toward their individual goals for a minimum of 4 wk. Control participants were on a wait list. *Outcome Measure* FIMBA: Ability to perform living skills and orientation and mobility skills at posttest.	The intervention group had significantly greater gains in living skills performance but not in orientation and mobility skills.	No psychometric properties were reported for the FIMBA. The outcome assessor was not blinded to group assignment.

Author/Year	Study Objectives	Level/Design/Participants	Intervention and Outcome Measures	Results	Limitations
Reeves et al. (2004) http://dx.doi.org/10.1136/bjo.2003.037457	To determine the effectiveness of an enhanced low vision rehabilitation model	Level I—Randomized control trial. *Participants* N = 194 participants with AMD and visual acuity < 6/18 Intervention group n = 64 Usual-care attention control group n = 70 Usual-care group n = 60 Median age = 81 yr	*Intervention* All three groups received conventional low vision rehabilitation in the clinic. The intervention group received 3 additional home visits by a rehabilitation practitioner to address the use of low vision aids, vision-enhancing strategies, and environmental modification. The usual-care attention control group received additional home visits from a community care worker. The usual-care group did not receive any home visits. *Outcome Measures* • Task performance test at 12-mo follow-up: Read 2 grocery items and 1 medicine bottle • Selected items on MLVQ: Restriction in daily activities at 12-mo follow-up.	Adding additional home-based low vision rehabilitation to the conventional rehabilitation did not result in better outcomes than the conventional rehabilitation program alone.	The researchers did not adjust for the progress of the eye condition in the analysis. Delivery of the home-based low vision rehabilitation program was not standard across the intervention group. The outcome assessment appeared to lack responsiveness. Most items in the MLVQ are reading tasks. No outcome assessment was done immediately after the intervention.
Scanlan & Cuddeford (2004)	To determine the effectiveness of a low vision service	Level I—Randomized control trial. *Participants* N = 64 participants with AMD and visual acuity < 20/60 Intervention group n = 32 Control group n = 32 Mean age = 81 yr	*Intervention* The intervention group received five 1-hr training sessions on the use of low vision assistive devices and compensation skills from a rehabilitation worker. The control group received only one 1-hr training session. *Outcome Measure* NEI VFQ–25 at 12 wk.	The intervention group showed significantly more improvement than the control group at 12 wk.	The NEI VFQ–25 was not administered immediately after the intervention.

(Continued)

Table D.1. Summary of Evidence on Interventions to Improve Performance of Daily Activities at Home for Older Adults With Low Vision *(Cont.)*

Author/Year[a]	Study Objectives	Level/Design/Participants[b]	Intervention and Outcome Measures	Results	Study Limitations
Smith et al. (2005)	To determine the effectiveness of custom prism spectacles	Level I—Randomized control trial. *Participants* N = 225 participants with AMD and visual acuity < 6/18 Custom prisms group n = 70 Standard prisms group n = 75 Nonprism specials group n = 80	*Intervention* All participants wore experimental spectacles at home for 3 mo. Participants wore prescribed custom bilateral prisms, prescribed standard bilateral prisms, or nonprism spectacles. *Outcome Measures* • NEI VFQ–25 at 3 mo • MLVAI: Performance in 16 ADLs (Part 1) and self-assessment in 9 ADLs (Part 2) at 3 mo.	No differences were found among groups.	Some participants may have compensated for vision loss with an eccentric viewing strategy.
http://dx.doi.org/10.1001/archopht.123.8.1042		Age range = 76–86 yr			
Stelmack et al. (2008, 2007)	To evaluate the effectiveness of a Veterans Affairs low vision intervention program	Level I—Randomized control trial. *Participants* N = 126 veterans with low vision and visual acuity < 20/100 Intervention group n = 64 Control group n = 62 Mean age = 79 yr	*Intervention* The intervention group received low vision devices, 5 weekly clinic sessions, and 1 home session. All sessions were provided by a low vision therapist who taught strategies to enhance remaining vision and the use of devices. The home session included environmental adaptation and assistance in setting up low vision devices. The control group did not receive any low vision intervention but did receive a bimonthly phone call from the therapist to prevent attrition. *Outcome Measure* VA LV VFQ–48: A questionnaire on daily activities related to reading, mobility, visual information processing, and visual-guided motor behavior at 4 mo and 1 yr.	The intervention group significantly improved compared with the control group at both follow-ups.	The sample was homogeneous, mostly male and White. No outcome assessment was done immediately after the intervention.
http://dx.doi.org/10.1001/archopht.126.5.608 http://dx.doi.org/10.1016/j.apmr.2007.03.025					

Vukicevic & Fitzmaurice (2009)	To evaluate the effectiveness of eccentric viewing	Level II—Quasi-experimental design. *Participants* $N = 48$ participants with AMD and visual acuity $< 20/200$ Intervention group $n = 24$ Attention control group $n = 24$ Mean age = 82 yr	*Intervention* The intervention group received 8 weekly sessions of eccentric viewing training at home from the researcher. The attention control group received weekly telephone calls from the researcher. *Outcome Measure* MLVAI Part 2: Self-assessed performance in 9 ADLs at 8 wk.	Significant improvement on ADLs was found in the intervention group. The same researcher provided training in both groups and collected data.

Note. ADLs = activities of daily living; AMD = age-related macular degeneration; FAQ = Functional Assessment Questionnaire; FIMBA = Functional Independence Measure for Blind Adults; FVPT = Functional Vision Performance Test; IADLs = instrumental activities of daily living; IVI = Impact of Vision Impairment; LVQOL = Low Vision Quality of Life questionnaire; MAI = Multilevel Assessment Instrument; MLVAI = Melbourne Low-Vision Assessment Instrument; MLVQ = Manchester Low Vision Questionnaire; NEI VFQ–25 = 25-item National Eye Institute Visual Functioning Questionnaire; VA LV VFQ–48 = Veteran Affairs Low Vision Visual Functioning Questionnaire–48.

[a]If multiple publications are from the same research study or program, the study listed first is the most recent, reported the outcomes most relevant to this review, or reported the highest level of evidence; other citations to the same study follow in parentheses.

[b]Only the number of participants who completed the study is reported in the table.

[c]Although the study used a two-group research design, we determined the level of evidence on the basis of the reviewed outcome, which was a pretest–posttest measure without group comparison.

Suggested citation: Liu, C.-J., Brost, M. A., Horton, V. E., Kenyon, S. B., & Mears, K. E. (2013). Occupational therapy interventions to improve performance of daily activities at home for older adults with low vision: A systematic review (Suppl. Table 1). *American Journal of Occupational Therapy, 67,* 279–287. http://dx.doi.org/10.5014/ajot.005512

Table D.2. Summary of Evidence on Interventions to Improve Reading Ability of Older Adults With Low Vision

Author/Year	Study Objectives	Level/Design/ Participants	Intervention and Outcome Measures	Results	Study Limitations
Theme 1: Effectiveness of Low Vision Devices					
Nguyen et al. (2009) http://dx.doi.org/10.1111/j.1755-3768.2008.01423.x	To determine the effects of LVDs on the reading ability of people with AMD	Level III—One-group, nonrandomized study with a pretest–posttest design; data collected retrospectively. *Participants* N = 530 participants in different stages of AMD Mean age = 82 yr; 73% were 75–90 yr old	*Intervention* First, participants read a passage of text (similar to newspaper print) without the use of LVDs. Then they were prescribed an appropriate LVD, trained in its use, and required to practice reading with the device for ≥ 30 min. They then read another passage of text while using the LVD. *Outcome Measure* Reading speed (wpm).	At pretest, only 16% of participants could read without a LVD; at posttest, 94% were able to read with a LVD. Of participants, 58% achieved reading ability with an optical visual aid, and 42% required electronic magnification (i.e., CCTV). Mean reading speed significantly from 16 wpm without LVDs to 72 wpm using LVDs.	The article did not report who carried out the intervention or in which the setting the intervention was conducted. No control group was used.
Theme 2: Comparison of Optical and Electronic Magnifying Devices					
Goodrich & Kirby (2001)	To compare the effects of 3 LVDs—a stand CCTV, a hand-held CCTV, and a prescribed optical device—on reading speed, reading duration, and participant preference	Level I—Within-participant design; participants served as their own controls. *Participants* N = 22 veterans (20 men and 2 women) with severe low vision Age range: 53–87; Mean age = 73.3 yr	*Intervention* Participants received eccentric viewing training and then were provided 5 sessions of formal reading rehabilitation training in the use of 3 LVDs. They then read paragraphs with each device and answered questions regarding device preference. *Outcome Measures* • Reading speed (wpm), duration (min), and comprehension • Reading productivity (words per sitting; reading speed × duration).	Reading speed, duration, and productivity were greater with CCTVs than with prescribed optical devices. Optical devices required lower magnification than CCTVs, but closer working distances. For participants with 20/200 acuity or greater, stand-mounted CCTVs resulted in the greatest reading speeds. For those with < 20/200 acuity, hand-held CCTVs produced highest reading speeds. Participants preferred the stand-mounted CCTV, reporting that it was easiest to use, more convenient for lengthy reading, and most likely to be purchased considering its out-of-pocket expense. For short reading, 50% preferred the hand-held CCTV and 50% preferred the stand-mounted CCTV.	Training in the use of low vision assistive devices was provided by four different instructors, which may have affected the uniformity of the intervention across participants; however, all instructors had extensive previous experience in clinical instruction, and no indication was found of systematic differences between instructors.

Study	Purpose	Design/Participants	Intervention/Outcome Measures	Results	Comments
Peterson et al. (2003) http://dx.doi.org/10.1016/S0002-9394(03)00567-1	To determine the advantages of various EVES compared with the participant's own optical magnifier in improving objective near-task performance and to analyze the effect of previous optical and EVES experience on reading speed and task performance	Level I—Within-patient design. *Participants* $N = 70$ participants (35 male and 35 female) with low vision; specific diagnoses included AMD ($n = 40$ participants), vascular retinopathy ($n = 11$), diabetic retinopathy ($n = 9$), corneal conditions ($n = 6$), and open-angle glaucoma ($n = 4$) Mean age = 70 yr	*Intervention* In a hospital ophthalmology low vision clinic, participants received an explanation, demonstration, and 2-min training regarding the use of a personal optical magnifier, a mouse-based EVES with monitor viewing, a mouse-based EVES with HMD viewing, and a stand-based EVES with monitor viewing. Each participant then completed 4 tasks using the 4 devices. *Outcome Measures* • Reading speed and acuity using MNRead Acuity Charts (Precision Vision, LaSalle, IL) adapted for the study • Column tracking (tracking from one print column to the next) • Map tracking (following a map route and locating a specific feature) • Label identification (identifying information on a medicine bottle) • Perception of ease of use of each magnifier and difficulty of each test on a 0–5 scale.	Previous experience with magnifiers or EVESs did not significantly influence task performance. Reading speeds were fastest using the stand EVES, followed by the mouse EVES with HDM viewing and personal optical magnifiers. Personal optical magnifiers resulted in faster completion rates for column tracking than the other magnifiers. Personal optical magnifiers and stand EVESs with monitor viewing resulted in faster completion rates for map tracking than the other magnifiers. Personal optical magnifiers and stand or mouse EVESs with monitor viewing produced the fastest completion rates for label identification. Participants rated the stand EVES with monitor viewing easiest to use, followed by the mouse EVES with HMD viewing. The mouse EVES with HMD viewing and personal optical magnifiers were rated at similar difficulty levels. In general, participants rated a stand EVES and a mouse EVES similarly in ease of use. EVES may be easier to use, but optical magnification also can provide the magnification and speed needed for many ADLs.	The article did not identify who carried out the intervention. The participants received only 2 min of training for each EVES, for many their first exposure to and use of an EVES; this duration may have been insufficient for the participants to become familiar with the EVES.

(Continued)

Table D.2. Summary of Evidence on Interventions to Improve Reading Ability of Older Adults With Low Vision *(Cont.)*

Author/Year	Study Objectives	Level/Design/Participants	Intervention and Outcome Measures	Results	Study Limitations
			Theme 3: Effectiveness of Low Vision Rehabilitation Programs That Include Occupational Therapy		
Eklund et al. (2008)	To compare the effects of a health promotion program with an individual program on ADL dependence of older adults with AMD	Level I—Randomized control trial. *Participants* *N* = 131 participants with AMD Health promotion group *n* = 62 Individual (control) group *n* = 69 Age = 65+	*Intervention* The health promotion program was a group intervention led by occupational therapists. Groups met for one 2-hr session per wk for 8 wk. Other professionals (ophthalmologist, optician, low vision therapist, lighting expert) also provided information. The individual program was considered standard care and consisted of one or two 1-hr individual sessions with an occupational therapist trained in low vision. *Outcome Measure* Level of dependence in ADLs measured on a scale ranging from 0 (*independent*) to 9 (*dependent*).	At 28-mo follow-up, participants in the individual group were more dependent in ADLs than participants in the health promotion group. Participants in the health promotion group maintained their current level of function in ADLs at follow-up.	Many participants were lost between recruiting and follow-up. The evaluators were not blinded to which intervention the participants had received.

http://dx.doi.org/10.1080/11038120701442963

Author/Year	Study Objectives	Level/Design/Participants	Intervention and Outcome Measures	Results	Study Limitations
Markowitz et al. (2008)	To determine the effects of low vision rehabilitation on the ability of older adults with low vision to read standard medication labels	Level III—Prospective, nonrandomized interventional case series design. *Participants* *N* = 57 participants (61% female, 31% male) with AMD (78%), glaucoma (9%), and other conditions (13%) Age range = 49–95 yr; Median age = 80 yr	*Intervention* Participants were instructed in the assembly, maintenance, and use of prescribed LVDs (high-powered reading glasses, magnifiers, electronic magnification). Occupational therapists trained participants to use large-print materials, proper reading distances, adequate illumination, and strategies for viewing curved surfaces. *Outcome Measure* Ability to read standard labels on prescription medication bottles, rated on a 0–2 scale.	At initial evaluation, 58% of participants were unable to identify information on their prescribed medications (0 on the scale). 40% were partially able to read the information (1 on the scale), and 2% were able to read the information (2 on the scale). At discharge, 94% of participants rated their ability as 2, 4% rated their ability as 1, and 2% rated their ability as 0, indicating a major improvement in ability to read medication labels after LVD prescription and training.	The study did not incorporate nonvisual techniques to read the labels, which is an alternative for those who cannot visually read labels.

Author/Year	Study Objectives	Level/Design and Participants	Intervention and Outcome Measures	Results	Study Limitations
McCabe et al. (2000)	To determine whether vision rehabilitation involving optometry, occupational therapy, and social work services improved the functional ability of older adults with low vision	Level I—Randomized control trial. *Participants* $N = 97$; diagnoses included macular degeneration (64%), diabetic retinopathy (13%), other retinal diseases (12%), optic neuropathy (7%), glaucoma (3%), and cataracts (1%). Individual protocol $n = 48$ Family protocol $n = 49$ 25 participants withdrew from the study, leaving a final N of 72.	*Intervention* Participants received the standard vision rehabilitation of training in the use of prescribed optical and nonoptical devices, instruction in adaptive techniques, adjustment counseling, or all of these. The occupational therapist trained participants to use optical and nonoptical devices and adaptive techniques to maximize visual capacities. *Outcome Measures* • Modified FAQ: Gains in functional activity • FVPT: Speed and accuracy in spot-reading tasks, short-term text reading, identification of paper currency, and clock reading.	Participants experienced a significant gain in visual capacity, as measured by the FVPT, and a significant decrease in dependency and self-reported difficulty in performing tasks, as measured by the FAQ. Additionally, on the FAQ, participants reported a significant decrease in difficulty performing tasks. These findings indicate that vision rehabilitation intervention involving services from an optometrist, an occupational therapist, and a social worker is effective in improving performance of visual tasks.	The table providing participant characteristics included the participants who dropped out and were not included in the results.

http://dx.doi.org/10.1076/opep.7.4.259.4173   Mean age = 69 yr

Theme 4: Effectiveness of Low Vision Rehabilitation Programs That Do Not Include Occupational Therapy Services

Author/Year	Study Objectives	Level/Design and Participants	Intervention and Outcome Measures	Results	Study Limitations
Scanlan & Cuddeford (2004)	To determine the effectiveness of a low vision rehabilitation program for older adults with AMD that included an extended period of education in the use of LVDs	Level I—Randomized control trial. *Participants* $N = 64$ Experimental group $n = 32$ Control group $n = 32$ Mean age = 81 yr	*Intervention* The experimental group received extensive training in reading techniques such as eccentric viewing and in the correction of skills. The instructor also assigned progressively more difficult reading activities. *Control* The control group received a 1-hr traditional training session. *Outcome Measures* • Pepper Visual Skills for Reading Test: Reading speed and accuracy • NEI VFQ–25: Health-related quality of life.	The experimental group significantly improved in reading speed and accuracy compared with the control group, and the benefits of the extended training sessions were maintained over time. The experimental group indicated significantly greater improvement in perceived quality of life compared with the control group after completion of the extended training period.	The participants were recruited from a limited geographic area. No follow-up was done.

(Continued)

Table D.2. Summary of Evidence on Interventions to Improve Reading Ability of Older Adults With Low Vision (*Cont.*)

Author/Year	Study Objectives	Level/Design/ Participants	Intervention and Outcome Measures	Results	Study Limitations
Stelmack et al. (2008)	To examine the effectiveness of an outpatient low vision rehabilitation program, the Low Vision Intervention Trial (LOVIT), on reading performance and visual ability	Level 1—Multicenter Randomized control trial. *Participants* N = 126 with diagnoses of AMD, macular dystrophy, macular hole, and inflammatory disease of the macula Treatment group n = 64 Control group n = 62 Nine participants in the treatment group dropped out before completion, leaving 55 in the treatment group and 117 in the entire study. Mean age = 79 yr	*Intervention* The treatment group received a low vision examination, education, LVD prescription, 6 weekly low vision therapy sessions (1 completed at home), and homework. Low vision therapy addressed visual ability, including near spot checking, table reading, long-duration reading, spot checking at far and intermediate distances, glare control, and long-duration distance viewing. The control group received treatment after a delay of 4 mo (typical amount of time veterans spend on a waiting list). They received 2 telephone calls per month. *Outcome Measure* Low Vision Visual Functioning Questionnaire–48: Reading ability.	Participants in the treatment group reported significant improvement in visual reading ability from baseline to the 4-mo follow-up compared with the control group. Participants in the control group showed a slight decrease in visual reading from baseline to the 4-mo follow-up. This common low vision rehabilitation intervention model was effective in improving visual reading ability for people with low vision.	Because this study did not use a placebo for the control group, the authors indicated they could not rule out a Hawthorne effect in which participants change their behavior simply because they are aware they are being studied.
http://dx.doi.org/10.1001/archopht.126.5.608					

Theme 5: Effectiveness of Nonoptical Devices

| Bowers, Meek, & Stewart (2001) | To compare an objectively determined optimal illumination with preferred illumination on reading performance in older adults with AMD | Level 1—Randomized control trial; participants acted as their own controls. *Participants* N = 20 participants with AMD Age range = 60–85 yr | *Intervention* In a clinic, participants binocularly read MNRead Acuity Charts without using LVDs at 6 levels of task illumination (50, 300, 600, 1,000, 2,000, and 5,000 lux) presented in random order. *Outcome Measures* • Reading speed (wpm) • Optimal illumination level • Preferred illumination level. | Reading speed improved the most between the illumination levels of 50 lux and 2,000 lux. Compared with normal room illumination (600 lux) or with typical home lighting (50 lux), reading rate and acuity were best at optimal illumination. Maximum reading rate improved by 36 wpm between 50 and 5,000 lux. Most participants (70%) preferred a lower level of illumination than that at which they optimally performed. | The article did not indicate who carried out the intervention. |
| http://dx.doi.org/10.1111/j.1444-0938.2001.tb04957.x | | | | | |

Eperjesi et al. (2007)	To compare 4 commonly used lamps of varying radiance on the reading performance of older adults with either age-related maculopathy or nonexudative AMD	Level I—Prospective Randomized control trial; participants acted as their own controls. *Participants* N = 13 participants with either AMD or age-related maculopathy Age range = 55–82; Mean age = 69 yr	*Intervention* At a 40-cm reading distance and an illumination level of 2,000 lux, participants read from a MNRead card (to establish their threshold print size) under 4 lamps: standard (clear envelope) incandescent, daylight simulation (blue tint envelope) incandescent, halogen incandescent, and compact cool white fluorescent. *Outcome Measure* Reading speed (wpm).	No significant difference was found between any of the lamps and their effects on reading performance. This research adds to the body of evidence indicating that the type of light source is not a critical factor when recommending task lighting to older adults with low vision.	The sample size was small, and only 2 diagnoses were represented. Some participants' visual acuity was adequate. The authors used the same intervention illumination level of 2,000 lux for all participants rather than determine each participant's optimum illumination level.
Kabanarou & Rubin (2006)	To compare the effects of binocular vs. monocular viewing on reading performance in participants with bilateral AMD	Level I—One-group, within-subjects study. *Participants* N = 22 diagnosed with bilateral late-stage AMD Mean age = 81 yr	*Intervention* Participants read aloud with both eyes, then with their better eye while the other eye was occluded. Text size was adjusted for each task on the basis of acuity. *Outcome Measure* Reading speed (wpm).	Participants read faster when using binocular viewing compared with monocular viewing; however, the difference was not significant. Reading speed in the better eye is a good predictor of binocular reading speed. No significant difference was found in binocular vs. monocular reading performance.	If the participants read a sentence incorrectly, it was excluded from analysis unless the participant corrected the error. Inaccurately read sentences were not included in the data analysis, which may have falsely enhanced the positive findings.

http://dx.doi.org/10.1097/01.opx.0000238642.65218.64

(Continued)

Table D.2. Summary of Evidence on Interventions to Improve Reading Ability of Older Adults With Low Vision (*Cont.*)

Author/Year	Study Objectives	Level/Design/ Participants	Intervention and Outcome Measures	Results	Study Limitations
Russell-Minda et al. (2007)	To review available evidence regarding the attributes of type-faces on text legibility for people with low vision	Level 1—Systematic review (mainly Level II articles). *Inclusion criteria:* Articles were written in English and addressed legibility and attributes of French-language typefaces for people with low vision who desire to read. All types of low vision diagno-ses and study designs were included. Issues regarding international guidelines or standards for legibility of type-faces for print-disabled people were included. Studies of computer accessibility were excluded.	*Intervention* Two of the authors separately reviewed and rated the abstracts on the basis of level of evidence. Studies were primarily nonrandomized or experimental or were unpublished. *Outcome Measure* Attributes of typefaces influencing text legibility for people with low vision.	The review, which included 18 studies, was inconclusive regarding serifs, yet there may be a subjective preference for sans serif fonts. Fonts such as Verdana, Helvetica, Arial, and Adsans may be more readable than Times New Roman. Boldface, sans serif typefaces that are at least 12 points in size are preferred for reading medication information on both rounded and flat surfaces. Font size should be at least 16–18 points, although no consensus exists on the best font size for low vision materials. Print size must be larger when reading in the periphery than with central vision.	The authors did not review research on optimal typefaces and print size associated with computer accessibility.

Author/Year	Study Objectives, Level, and Design	Intervention and Outcome Measures	Results	Study Limitations
Vukicevic & Fitzmaurice (2005) http://dx.doi.org/10.1080/13388235050037762	To determine the effects of eccentric viewing and magnification interventions on the ability of older adults with AMD to perform ADLs Level I—Randomized control trial. *Participants* N = 58 participants (39 women and 19 men) with AMD with an absolute scotoma Eccentric viewing n = 22 Combination n = 12 Magnification n = 12 No intervention n = 12 Age range = 60–96; Mean age = 82 yr	*Intervention* *Eccentric viewing group:* Trained in eccentric viewing using the EccVue computer program over 8 weekly sessions. *Combination group:* Trained in eccentric viewing and instructed in magnification use. *Magnification group:* Instructed in the use of magnification. *No-intervention group:* Received a weekly phone call of ≤ 15 min over 8 wk. *Outcome Measures* • Near print size determined with the Bailey–Lovie Reading Card • Performance of ADLs using the Melbourne Low Vision ADL Index Part A, ability to perform high-acuity daily tasks, and Part B, ability to perform lower acuity daily tasks.	Participants in each experimental group significantly improved their near print size scores. The eccentric viewing and combination groups maintained these scores at the follow-up. All 3 experimental groups significantly improved their Part A scores on the Melbourne Low Vision ADL Index. The eccentric viewing and combination groups improved significantly in Part B scores. The majority of participants in the eccentric viewing (77%) and combination (75%) groups reported the intervention had been helpful, compared with 58% of the magnification group and 0% of the no-intervention group. Eccentric viewing training along with magnification training was recommended.	Although the study found improvements in ability to perform ADLs with use of eccentric viewing and magnification, the authors did not specify what ADLs they assessed or which improved. Therefore, it is impossible to tell whether the increase in ability can be attributed to tasks that involved reading.

Table D.3. Summary of Evidence on Low Vision Interventions to Promote Driving and Community Mobility for Older Adults With Low Vision

Author	Study Objectives	Level/Design/Participants	Intervention and Outcome Measures	Results	Study Limitations
			Driving Simulation		
Akinwuntan et al. (2005)	To determine the effectiveness of simulator-based training on driving performance and safety poststroke	Level I—Randomized control trial. *Participants* N = 73 participants with first stroke age < 75 yr who were able to legally drive before the stroke (~25% had visual field loss)	*Intervention* Regular hospital rehabilitation programming and driver simulator training, 15 hr over 5 wk. *Control* Driving-related cognitive tasks. *Outcome Measures* • Fitness-to-drive evaluation classification (unfit to drive, temporarily unfit to drive, fit to drive) • On-road test performance.	Of intervention participants who completed the follow-up assessment, 73% passed and could legally resume driving compared with only 42% of control participants ($p = .03$). Simulator outcomes showed significant reductions in collisions, pedestrian hits, and total faults (all $ps < .001$) for the intervention group.	The authors provided limited description of the simulator protocol and of the measure for determining fitness to drive, limiting reproducibility. Only about 25% of participants were reported to have visual field loss; their outcomes were not differentiated from those of participants with no visual field loss. No significant difference was found between the intervention and control groups regarding visual field loss. Simulated outcomes were not compared with on-road measures, so the study lacks ecological validity.

http://dx.doi.org/10.1212/01.wnl.0000171749.71919.fa

Author	Study Objectives	Level/Design/Participants	Intervention and Outcome Measures	Results	Study Limitations
			Multidisciplinary Low Vision Rehabilitation		
Lamoureux et al. (2007)	To evaluate the effectiveness of a multidisciplinary low vision rehabilitation program on quality of life	Level III—Before-and-after design. *Participants* N = 192 participants with AMD Mean age = 80.3 ± 13.1 yr	*Intervention* Multidisciplinary low vision services to help participants use their remaining vision, improve participation in daily living, and improve quality of life after an initial assessment at a low vision clinic with a member of the multidisciplinary team usually made up of occupational therapy, orientation and mobility, orthoptics, and welfare specialists. Devices and rehabilitation program provided for ≤ 6 mo.	Participants showed significant improvements on all IVI subscales except the Mobility and Independence subscale. The highest effect size was obtained for the Emotional Well-Being subscale.	Not all participants took advantage of occupational therapy or O&M services (n = 48 participants). Comorbidities may have led to decreased O&M scores. No control group was used. The discussion of the IVI instrument and Independence subscale lacks detail on how the items contribute to the construct of community mobility.

Outcome Measures

Impact of Visual Impairment (IVI): Self-reported restriction of participation in daily living activities on the basis of ability to read and access information and emotional well-being and level of mobility and independence.

http://dx.doi.org/10.1167/iovs.06-0610

Driver Education Programs

| Owsley et al. (2004) | To evaluate the efficacy of a program that teaches older drivers at high risk for crash involvement and motivated to remain behind the wheel the effects of their functional deficits on driving skills and compensatory strategies such as self-regulation | Level I—Randomized control trial.

Participants
$N = 403$ licensed drivers with visual impairment ages ≥ 60 yr in the Birmingham, Alabama, area who had been the driver in a crash in the prior yr and had a Mini-Mental State Examination score of ≥ 23 | *Intervention*
Usual care (comprehensive examination by an optometrist; discussion with an eye care specialist of the impact of any diagnosed visual impairment on activities of daily living, including driving) plus 2 educational sessions that included an initial 2-hr visit followed by a booster session 1 mo later.

Control
Usual care alone.

Outcome Measures
• Crash involvement during 2-yr follow-up
• Average weekly mileage and average days, trips, and places driven per wk measured at 6-, 12-, 18-, and 24-mo interviews. | At 2-yr follow-up, no difference was found in crash rates between the two groups. Both groups reported decreases in mileage driven, with a more significant decrease ($p = .02$) occurring in the intervention group.

For both driving avoidance and self-regulation scores, after baseline equivalence, the intervention group had significantly higher scores than the usual-care group at each follow-up visit (both $ps < .001$). | Outcomes for the 2-yr follow-up were self-reported.

Two intervention sessions may not have been enough to change behaviors for the long term.

The education provided may have made participants overconfident in their ability to continue driving. |

http://dx.doi.org/10.1016/j.amepre.2003.12.005

(Continued)

Table D.3. Summary of Evidence on Low Vision Interventions to Promote Driving and Community Mobility for Older Adults With Low Vision (Cont.)

Author	Study Objectives	Level/Design/Participants	Intervention and Outcome Measures	Results	Study Limitations
Stalvey & Owsley (2003)	To evaluate the efficacy of a theory-based intervention for high-risk older drivers	Level I—Randomized control trial. *Participants* N = 365 participants ages ≥ 60 yr who were legally licensed to drive in Alabama, who had visual acuity of 20/30 to 20/60 or visual processing deficits, and who had a high level of driving exposure and a history of crash involvement Mean age = 74 yr	*Intervention* Usual care plus 2 educational sessions that included an initial 2-hr visit followed by a booster session 1 mo later. *Control* Usual care. *Outcome Measure* Driver Perceptions and Practices Questionnaire before and after interventions.	Participants in the educational program reported a significantly greater level of perceived vision impairment and understanding about its impact on driving and a significantly higher number of perceived benefits of self-regulation.	Outcomes for the 2-yr follow-up were self-reported. Two intervention sessions may not have been enough to change behaviors for the long term. The education provided may have made participants overconfident in their ability to continue driving.
Low Vision Devices (Bioptics and Prisms)					
Bowers et al. (2005)	To determine participants' perceived ability to continue driving safely after receiving bioptic telescope training	Level III—Cross-sectional survey study design. *Participants* N = 58 drivers with visual impairments who had recent experience in driving with a bioptic telescope and who used or were trained to use bioptics during driving within the past 3 yr Age range = 17–86 yr	*Intervention* No intervention; previous participation in driver training with the use of bioptics. *Outcome Measures* Driving Habits Questionnaire (DHQ), supplemented with questions specific to driving with bioptic telescopes.	83% of participants reported driving themselves. 72% rated their driving as above average. 84% reported driving with the general flow of traffic. 88% were moderately or very confident using bioptics while driving. Of participants age 65 and younger, 40% reported having no access to public transportation in their area, 90% were employed, and 85% drove to work. 12% reported 1 crash in the previous 12 mo.	Several participants were referred to physicians to assist in answering questions on the DHQ. Participants' age range of 17–86 limits generalizability to the older population. Outcomes were not differentiated by age. No details were provided on dosage of driver training with bioptics (time, intensity, duration).

http://dx.doi.org/10.1167/iovs.04-0271

Study	Design/Participants	Intervention and Outcome Measures	Results	Limitations
Szlyk et al. (1998)	Level II—Crossover design. *Participants* N = 15 Mean age = 45.2 yr; Age range = 27–67 yr	*Intervention* O&M training, 4 weekly 3-hr sessions; driving training, 8 weekly 2-hr sessions. *Outcome Measures* *O&M assessment:* • Visual skill tasks in the domains of recognition, peripheral detection, scanning, tracking, and mobility (outdoor activities; e.g., crossing intersections). *Driving assessment:* • Visual skill tasks in the domains of recognition, peripheral detection, scanning, tracking, visual memory, and mobility (simulator and on-road skills; e.g., number of accidents, brake response time).	No statistically significant differences were found between groups when comparing distribution of scores for improvement. Overall improvement for both groups averaged 37.3%. Mobility scores improved 46.4%. Of participants, 86% were satisfied or extremely satisfied with bioptics.	The small sample size limits power and generalizability. Only 1 of the 15 participants was > 65 yr old. No breakdown was reported for skills specific to O&M or driving, making it difficult to attribute change to outdoor mobility or driving training. No reference was made to crash or on-road performance outcomes (pass vs. fail). Psychometric characteristics of the outcome measures were not reported.
To test the effectiveness of a bioptic, peripheral vision–enhancement lens in participants with retinitis pigmentosa, choroidemia, and Usher's syndrome Type II				

http://dx.doi.org/10.1097/00006324-199807000-00021

Study	Design/Participants	Intervention and Outcome Measures	Results	Limitations
Szlyk et al. (2000)	Level I—Randomized control trial. *Participants* N = 25 participants (13 male and 12 female) with central vision loss Age range = 16–78 yr	*Intervention* • *Training groups:* O&M training, 4 weekly 3-hr sessions, and driving training, 8 weekly 2-hr sessions • *Control groups:* (1) delayed training and (2) no training. *Outcome Measures* • O&M assessment: Visual skill tasks in the domains of recognition, peripheral detection, scanning, tracking, and mobility (outdoor activities; e.g., crossing intersections) • Driving assessment: Visual skill tasks in the domains of recognition, peripheral detection, scanning, tracking, visual memory, and mobility (simulator and on-road skills; e.g., number of accidents, brake response time).	Training groups demonstrated improved visual skills in the domains of recognition, peripheral detection, and scanning. No significant improvement was found in the domains of mobility, tracking, and visual memory; however, when driving skills were compared separately, a significant difference was found between the trained and untrained groups ($p = .02$). 82% of participants were very satisfied or extremely satisfied with bioptics.	The small sample size limits power and generalizability. The low proportion (25%) of participants > 65 yr old limits generalizability to the older population. Driving-related skill improvement was noted, but no reference was made to crash or on-road performance outcomes (pass vs. fail). Limited detail was provided on how driving items and skills were quantified (possibly mixed domains). Psychometric characteristics of the outcome measures were not reported.
To evaluate a vision rehabilitation program aimed at training people with visual field loss to use a bioptic telescope to improve life skills, including driving				

(Continued)

Table D.3. Summary of Evidence on Low Vision Interventions to Promote Driving and Community Mobility for Older Adults With Low Vision (*Cont.*)

Author	Study Objectives	Level/Design/Participants	Intervention and Outcome Measures	Results	Study Limitations
Szlyk et al. (2005)	To compare the outcomes of orientation and mobility and driver training with Fresnel prisms and the Gottlieb Visual Field Awareness System (VFAS) for participants with homonymous hemianopsia To determine whether the participants continued to use the optical enhancement devices at 2-yr follow-up	Level II—Crossover, cohort design. *Participants* $N = 10$ men with hemianopsia Mean age = 52.3 yr; Age range = 16–74 yr	*Intervention* Lab and outdoor training with Fresnel or Gottlieb VFAS prisms, four 2- to 3-hr sessions; on-road training, eight 2-hr sessions. *Outcome Measures* • Outdoor functional assessment: Visual skill tasks in the domains of recognition, peripheral detection, scanning, tracking, and mobility (outdoor activities; e.g., crossing intersections) scored by a certified O&M specialist. • Driving skills assessment: Visual skill tasks in the domains of recognition, peripheral detection, scanning, tracking, visual memory, and mobility (simulator and on-road skills; e.g., number of accidents, brake response time).	Participants improved in all skill categories with both of the prism systems, ranging from 36% for mobility (Fresnel prisms) to 13% for recognition (Gottlieb VFAS). No statistically significant differences were found between types of prisms. 100% of the participants were at least satisfied with the prisms. At 2-yr follow-up, 3 of the 7 participants contacted were driving (43%); 2 (29%) were driving with the lenses.	Only 3 of the 10 participants were > 65 yr old, limiting generalization to the older population. Sample size was small. The description of the O&M training protocol lacks detail to facilitate reproducibility. Psychometric characteristics of the outcome measures were not reported. No breakdown was reported for items specific to outdoor mobility or driving in each skills domain, making it difficult to attribute change to outdoor mobility or driving training.

http://dx.doi.org/10.1111/j.1475-1313.2004.00265.x

Note. AMD = age-related macular degeneration; O&M = orientation and mobility.

This table is a product of AOTA's Evidence-Based Practice Project and the *American Journal of Occupational Therapy.* Copyright © 2013 by the American Occupational Therapy Association. It may be freely reproduced for personal use in clinical or educational settings as long as the source is cited. All other uses require written permission from the American Occupational Therapy Association. To apply, visit www.copyright.com.

Suggested citation: Justiss. M. D. (2013). Occupational therapy interventions to promote driving and community mobility for older adults with low vision: A systematic review (Suppl. Table 1). *American Journal of Occupational Therapy, 67,* 296–302. http://dx.doi.org/10.5014/ajot.005660

Table D.4. Summary of Evidence on Interventions to Improve Leisure and Social Participation for Older Adults With Low Vision

Author/Year	Study Objectives	Level/Design/Participants	Intervention and Outcome Measures	Results	Study Limitations
Brody et al. (1999) http://dx.doi.org/10.1007/BF02895965	To assess whether a self-management group intervention would increase engagement in activities and improve self-efficacy in people with vision loss	Level 1—Randomized control trial. *Participants* N = 92 participants with AMD Intervention group n = 44 Control group n = 48 Mean age = 79 yr; Age range = 65–91 yr *Interventionist* Not stated	*Intervention* Six weekly 2-hr self-management group sessions, including didactic presentations and problem-solving strategies with guided practice. *Control* Wait list; self-management intervention completed after the intervention group. *Outcome Measure* Health and Impact Questionnaire: General health and impact of macular degeneration on one's life, including participation in leisure activities.	Participants who provided activities data pre- and postintervention (n = 52) were significantly more likely to report engaging in gardening or landscaping (p < .001) and less likely to report going to movies (p < .001), attending cultural events (p = .006), or participating in religious observances (p < .001) after the intervention.	Time from assessment to intervention varied across participants, with an average of 3 mo; a change in baseline status could have occurred during this time.
Brunnström et al. (2004) http://dx.doi.org/10.1111/j.1475-1313.2004.00192.x	To determine the effect that adjusting task lighting in the living room has on the quality of life of older adults with low vision	Level 1—Randomized control trial. *Participants* N = 46 participants; macular degeneration (n = 28), retinitis pigmentosa (n = 2), glaucoma (n = 5), and other (n = 11) recruited from the Low Vision Clinic in Goteborg, Sweden Intervention group n = 24 Control group n = 22 Mean age = 76 yr; Age range = 20–90 yr *Interventionist* Occupational therapist	*Intervention* Light adjustments as needed in the kitchen, bathroom, and hall and task light adjustments around the living room reading area. *Control* Same treatment as the intervention group but no task light adjustments in the living room. *Outcome Measure* Perceived Quality of Life: Social participation factors including perception of loneliness, contact with relatives, and contact with others.	Participants in the intervention group experienced a significant improvement in social participation postintervention, whereas participants in the control group did not.	Information not reported includes group characteristics, reliability and validity of the outcome measure, and power of the sample size. The large range in ages of the participants may be a potential confounding factor.

(Continued)

Table D.4. Summary of Evidence on Interventions to Improve Leisure and Social Participation for Older Adults With Low Vision (*Cont.*)

Author/Year	Study Objectives	Level/Design/Participants	Intervention and Outcome Measures	Results	Study Limitations
Conrod & Overbury (1998)	To study the effects of perceptual training (PT) and individual (IC) and group (GC) psychosocial counseling on the adjustment of older adults living with vision loss	Level I—Randomized control trial. *Participants* $N = 99$ participants (49 with low vision [38 with AMD], 50 sighted controls) Mean age = 70 yr *Interventionist* Trained in administration of IC, GC, and PT manual	*Interventions* *PT:* Individualized training including scanning, peripheral viewing, and eye–hand coordination strategies *IC:* One-on-one instruction on 5 topics, including education, social participation, and community resources *GC:* Same instruction as the IC group but in a group setting. *Controls* • *Low vision:* Pre- and postintervention sessions only • *Sighted:* Single testing session. *Outcome Measures* • Activities questionnaire: Effect of vision loss on daily functioning, including shopping, socializing, and traveling • Expectations questionnaire: Expected performance on activities such as traveling, taking into account vision loss • Self-report questionnaire: Visual performance on routine tasks such as reading mail and writing letters.	No significant changes were observed on any of the measures related to leisure or social participation. Most participants in all 3 intervention groups resumed engagement in a meaningful activity that they had relinquished because of vision loss ($p = .08$). 77.8% of GC participants, 30.8% of IC participants, and 57.1% of PT participants reported initiating a new activity ($p = .09$).	Instructors were not blind to the participants' treatment status. Follow-up data were missing for 20 participants who could not be contacted.

		Intervention	Both groups showed an increase in perceived security at 4 mo in "reading an article in your newspaper," "threading a needle and sewing a button on," and "following the news on your TV."	The data collectors were not blind to the composition of the programs.
Dahlin Ivanoff et al. (2002)	To determine whether participation in a health education program would influence perceived security in the ability to engage in daily occupations for older adults with vision loss	Level I—Randomized control trial. *Participants* $N = 187$ participants with AMD recruited from low vision clinics at 2 university-affiliated hospitals in Sweden Health education group $n = 93$ Control group $n = 94$ Median age = 79 yr; Age range = 66–94 yr *Interventionist* Occupational therapist	Health education program in which an occupational therapist provided information and skills training in 8 occupational categories. *Control:* Individual intervention consisting of the standard care provided at the low vision clinics. *Outcome Measure* Questionnaire developed for the study: perceived security in performing 29 daily occupations in 7 areas.	Information such as participant characteristics, p values, and power of the sample size was not reported. The intervention group experienced significantly higher perceived security at 4 mo in "dialing on your phone," "finding your way in your local shop," "knowing your turn in the queue," and "writing a memo to yourself."
http://dx.doi.org/10.5014/ajot.56.3.322				
Elliott & Kuyk (1994)	To determine the impact of personal adjustment training on perception of quality of life	Level III—One group, nonrandomized design. *Participants* $N = 40$ veterans with vision loss Mean age = 64 yr; Age range = 36–85 yr *Interventionist* O&M specialist	*Intervention* Personal adjustment training for an average of 55 days at a residential program. *Outcome Measure* Survey developed for the study: functioning in the home environment, feelings of self-worth and self-confidence.	Significant improvements were seen in several areas, including social engagement, hobbies, and activities that use fine motor skills. The small sample size and lack of discussion of the intervention limit the ability to replicate the study and determine the causal factor of change.

(Continued)

Table D.4. Summary of Evidence on Interventions to Improve Leisure and Social Participation for Older Adults With Low Vision (*Cont.*)

Author/Year	Study Objectives	Level/Design/Participants	Intervention and Outcome Measures	Results	Study Limitations
Hinds et al. (2003)	To investigate the impact of an interdisciplinary low vision service on quality of life and participation in daily activities	Level III—Nonrandomized pretest–posttest. *Participants* $N = 71$ participants (68% with AMD) from two low vision clinics in Scotland Age: 78% > 71 yr; Age range: 34–86+ yr *Interventionists* Team including ophthalmologist, ophthalmic nurse, social worker, and rehabilitation worker	*Intervention* Interdisciplinary low vision service consisting of diagnosis, referral, blind or partially sighted registration, refraction and prescription of low vision aids, home visits, education, support, and counseling. *Outcome Measures* ▪ MLVQ: Performance, difficulty, and importance of 19 daily activities ▪ LVA measure: Use and helpfulness of prescribed LVAs during MLVQ tasks.	The number of people who reported reading ordinary print books, newsprint, or magazines increased significantly ($p = .049$). The number of people who reported reading large-print books and newspapers decreased significantly ($p = .015$). Nonsignificant improvements were seen in sewing and knitting, special hobbies, watching TV, and reading telephone numbers. 75% reported using prescribed LVAs during the past month while reading ordinary print books, newsprint, or magazines or watching TV. More than half found the LVAs useful for these tasks.	No control group was used.

http://dx.doi.org/10.1136/bjo.87.11.1391

La Grow (2004)	To determine the effectiveness of comprehensive low vision services vs. a mix of services currently available in promoting independent living skills for older adults with age-related vision loss	Level II—Nonrandomized controlled trial. *Participants* N = 186 participants recruited from 4 low vision clinics in New Zealand Intervention group n = 93 Control group n = 93 Mean age = 80.6 yr; Age range = 65–95 yr *Interventionist* Not stated	*Intervention* Vision examination; prescription for, loan of, and training in use of optical and nonoptical aids; follow-up and repeated visits if necessary. *Control* Typically available services—i.e, assessment and instruction in independent living skills, O&M, communication, and recreational and leisure activities. *Outcome Measure* Adapted version of Elliott and Kuyk's (1994) measure of functional and psychosocial outcomes of blind rehabilitation.	No significant differences were found between groups at posttest or follow-up.	The article does not provide results for the individual items in the outcome measure, so individual changes for each item of interest cannot be determined.
McCabe et al. (2000)	To determine whether vision rehabilitation increases patients' functional ability and whether involving families in intervention produces more successful outcomes	Level I—Randomized control trial. *Participants* N = 97 participants (64% with macular degeneration) Intervention group n = 49 Control group n = 48 Median age = 76 yr; Age range = 19–91 yr *Interventionists* Optometrist, occupational therapist, and social worker	*Intervention* *Family-focused care:* Standard vision rehabilitation (assessment; support services; and training in use of remaining vision, optical and nonoptical aids, and adaptive techniques) plus involvement of family members in all stages of intervention, education of family members about the ophthalmic condition and rehabilitation process, and instruction of family members in coping strategies to adapt to vision loss. *Control* *Individual care:* Standard vision rehabilitation. *Outcome Measure* FAQ: Visual function and overall well-being; relevant questions address travel and public transportation, sewing, doing a handicraft, and visiting friends.	A statistically significant decrease was found for both groups in dependency and difficulty in performing tasks. No significant differences were found between groups.	The sample size was not large enough to achieve statistical power. The results for individual items in the outcome measure were not reported.

http://dx.doi.org/10.1076/opep.7.4.259.4173

(Continued)

Table D.4. Summary of Evidence on Interventions to Improve Leisure and Social Participation for Older Adults With Low Vision (*Cont.*)

Author/Year	Study Objectives	Level/Design/Participants	Intervention and Outcome Measures	Results	Study Limitations
Pankow et al. (2004)	To determine whether a vision rehabilitation program would improve independent functioning in older adults with visual impairments	Level 1—Randomized control trial. *Participants* N = 30 participants (14 with AMD) Intervention group n = 15 Control group n = 15 Mean age = 75 yr; Age range = 65–90 yr *Interventionists* Occupational therapist, O&M specialist, rehabilitation teacher, and others	*Intervention* Customized treatment depending on participants' personal goals for rehabilitation consisting of rehabilitation teaching, O&M training, driving rehabilitation, and occupational therapy. *Control* Wait list for vision rehabilitation. *Outcome Measures* • FIMBA: Ability to perform living skills and O&M skills independently • Goal attainment: Participation in goals (e.g., hobbies, reading, cooking).	The treatment group had significantly higher scores than the control group on the FIMBA Living Skills Inventory. No significant difference was found in scores on the FIMBA Orientation and Mobility section. A significant difference between groups was found in goal attainment: 29 of 30 goals were attained in the intervention group, but only 1 of 30 goals was attained in the control group.	The sample size was small, and no mention was made of whether the study was adequately powered. Participants and evaluators were not blind to the composition of groups.
Reeves et al. (2004) http://dx.doi.org/10.1136/bjo.2003.037457	To determine whether people who received both supplementary home-based rehabilitation and conventional rehabilitation were better able to perform everyday activities than people who received only conventional rehabilitation	Level 1—Randomized control trial. *Participants* N = 226 participants with AMD recruited from the Manchester Royal Eye Hospital, England ELVR intervention group n = 75 CLVR control group n = 76 CELVR control group n = 75 Median age = 81 yr *Interventionist* Rehabilitation officer with training in vision rehabilitation and 5 yr of experience	*Intervention* ELVR: CLVR plus home-based low vision rehabilitation visits consisting of advice on, demonstration of, and supply of LVAs and support. *Controls* *CLVR group:* Setting and reappraisal of goals, demonstration of LVAs, discussion of ways to enhance vision, literature about diagnosis, and referrals and follow-up. *CELVR group:* CLVR and home-based visits during which participant and practitioner discuss problems and concerns and participation in daily and leisure activities. *Outcome Measure* MLVQ: Self-rated restriction in everyday activities because of visual impairment, duration of LVA use.	No significant differences were found between groups in the self-rated restriction score at 12 mo. No significant differences were found between groups in duration of LVA use.	Some patients were unmasked to the researchers during assessment.

Study	Study Objectives	Level/Design, Participants, Intervention, Control, Outcome Measures, and Interventionist	Results	Study Limitations
Rovner & Casten (2008) http://dx.doi.org/10.1097/IGP.0b013e3186b7342	To determine whether problem-solving treatment (PST) compared with usual care would reduce depression and prevent loss of participation in valued activities for people with AMD	**Level I**—Randomized control trial. *Participants* *N* = 206 participants with AMD and without clinical depression Intervention group *n* = 105 Control group *n* = 101 Age: > 64 yr *Interventionist* Nurse or counselor trained in PST	*Intervention* 6 in-home sessions of PST, an approach that teaches problem-solving skills through identifying the problem; goal setting; brainstorming, choosing, and implementing solutions; and evaluating outcomes. *Control* Usual care. *Outcome Measure* NEI VFQ–17: Difficulty participating in daily tasks such as reading the newspaper and engaging in hobbies, value of each activity.	Fewer participants in the intervention group gave up participation in valued activities (23.2% of intervention group vs. 37.4% of control group at 2 mo; 30.5% vs. 44.2% at 6 mo).	Limited information is provided about demographics (e.g., no mention of gender, race, mean age of group) and study procedures (e.g., no mention whether researchers were blind to groups). No explanation is provided of what "usual care" consisted of for the control group. Information is limited on whether the study controlled for additional services received by participants and other confounding factors.
Scanlan & Cuddeford (2004)	To determine the outcomes of a low vision service that provided an extended period of education in using low vision devices, specifically microscopes, for people with AMD	**Level I**—Randomized control trial. *Participants* *N* = 64 participants with AMD with best-corrected visual acuity in better eye of 20/60 to 20/400 recruited from new clients at the Canadian National Institute for the Blind Intervention group *n* = 32 Control group *n* = 32 Mean age = 81 yr; Age range = 65–89 yr *Interventionist* Vision rehabilitation nurse	*Intervention* Five 1-hr educational sessions by a vision rehabilitation nurse individualized to participant needs and focused on reading skills. *Control* 1-hr educational session on use of optical devices by a vision rehabilitation nurse. *Outcome Measure* NEI VFQ–25: Difficulty participating in daily tasks such as reading the newspaper and engaging in hobbies.	The NEI VFQ–25 showed a statistically significant difference between groups at Time 3 (follow-up at week 12), when the experimental group rated their eyesight as better, expressed less difficulty reading smaller print (newspapers, telephone books), expressed less difficulty seeing how others reacted to things they said, and perceived that they needed less help from others.	Sample size was small.

(Continued)

Table D.4. Summary of Evidence on Interventions to Improve Leisure and Social Participation for Older Adults With Low Vision *(Cont.)*

Author/Year	Study Objectives	Level/Design/Participants	Intervention and Outcome Measures	Results	Study Limitations
Shuttleworth et al. (1995) http://dx.doi.org/10.1136/bjo.79.8.719	To measure the effectiveness of an integrated low vision rehabilitation program using LVAs in improving function and satisfaction for people with vision loss over a 2-yr period	Level III—One-group longitudinal design. *Participants* *N* = 125 participants (47% with AMD) at study onset (111 at 1 yr, 75 at 2 yr) recruited from the Low Vision Clinic in South Devon, England Mean age = 76 yr *Interventionist* Orthoptist with 3 mo training in low vision rehabilitation	*Intervention* Functional assessment, individualized counseling, advice and training in use of LVAs and visual techniques, and referrals to social services; loan of most appropriate LVA to participants. *Outcome Measure* Questionnaire: Use of LVAs and satisfaction with low vision services.	Most participants used LVAs for near vision tasks, including reading correspondence (83% at 1 yr, 86% at 2 yr) and pleasure reading (73% and 64%). Some participants used LVAs for writing (39% at 1 yr and 25% at 2 yr) and hobbies (27% and 16%).	No control group was used to provide comparison data. Limited baseline data were presented.

Note. AMD = age-related macular degeneration; CELVR = control for additional contact time in enhanced low vision rehabilitation; CLVR = conventional low vision rehabilitation; ELVR = enhanced low vision rehabilitation; FAQ = Functional Assessment Questionnaire; FIMBA = Functional Independence Measure for Blind Adults; LVA = low vision aid; MLVQ = Manchester Low Vision Questionnaire; NEI VFQ–17 = 17-item National Eye Institute Visual Function Questionnaire; O&M = orientation and mobility.

This table is a product of AOTA's Evidence-Based Practice Project and the *American Journal of Occupational Therapy*. Copyright © 2013 by the American Occupational Therapy Association. It may be freely reproduced for personal use in clinical or educational settings as long as the source is cited. All other uses require written permission from the American Occupational Therapy Association. To apply, visit www.copyright.com.

Suggested citation: Berger, S., McAteer, J., Schreier, K., & Kaldenberg, J. (2013). Occupational therapy interventions to improve leisure and social participation for older adults with low vision: A systematic review (Suppl. Table 1). *American Journal of Occupational Therapy, 67,* 303–311. http://dx.doi.org/10.5014/ajot.005447

References

Accreditation Council for Occupational Therapy Education. (2012). 2011 Accreditation Council for Occupational Therapy Education (ACOTE®) standards. *American Journal of Occupational Therapy, 66,* S6–S74. http://dx.doi.org/10.5014/ajot.2012.66S6

Agency for Healthcare Research and Quality, U.S. Preventive Services Task Force. (2009). *Standard recommendation language.* Retrieved February 14, 2009, from http://www.uspreventiveservicestaskforce.org/uspstf.htm

Akinwuntan, A. E., De Weerdt, W., Feys, H., Pauwels, J., Baten, G., Arno, P., & Kiekens, C. (2005). Effect of simulator training on driving after stroke: A randomized controlled trial. *Neurology, 65,* 843–850. http://dx.doi.org/10.1212/01.wnl.0000171749.71919.fa

American Medical Association. (2012). *CPT 2013.* Chicago: Author.

American Occupational Therapy Association. (1979). Uniform terminology for occupational therapy. *Occupational Therapy News, 35,* 1–8.

American Occupational Therapy Association. (1989). Uniform terminology for occupational therapy (2nd ed.). *American Journal of Occupational Therapy, 43,* 808–815. http://dx.doi.org/10.5014/ajot.43.12.808

American Occupational Therapy Association. (1994). Uniform terminology for occupational therapy (3rd ed.). *American Journal of Occupational Therapy, 48,* 1047–1054. http://dx.doi.org/10.5014/ajot.48.11.1047

American Occupational Therapy Association. (2002). Occupational therapy practice framework: Domain and process. *American Journal of Occupational Therapy, 56,* 609–639. http://dx.doi.org/10.5014/ajot.56.6.609

American Occupational Therapy Association. (2006). Policy 1.44: Categories of occupational therapy personnel. In *Policy manual* (2011 ed., pp. 33–34). Bethesda, MD: Author.

American Occupational Therapy Association. (2008). Occupational therapy practice framework: Domain and process (2nd ed.). *American Journal of Occupational Therapy, 62,* 625–688. http://dx.doi.org/10.5014/ajot.62.6.625

American Occupational Therapy Association. (2009). Guidelines for supervision, roles and responsibilities during the delivery of therapy services. *American Journal of Occupational Therapy, 58,* 663–667. http://dx.doi.org/10.5014/ajot.63.6.797

American Occupational Therapy Association. (2010). Standards of practice for occupational therapy. *American Journal of Occupational Therapy, 64,* S106–S111. http://dx.doi.org/10.5014/ajot.2010.64S106

American Occupational Therapy Association. (2011). *AOTA's societal statement on health literacy. American Journal of Occupational Therapy, 65*(Suppl.), S78–S79. http://dx.doi.org/10.5014/ajot.2011.65S78

American Occupational Therapy Association. (2013). Guidelines for documentation of occupational therapy. *American Journal of Occupational Therapy, 67*(Suppl.).

Baldasare, J., Watson, G., Whittaker, S., & Miller-Shaffer, H. (1986). The development and evaluation of a reading test for low vision individuals with macular loss. *Journal of Visual Impairment and Blindness, 80,* 785–789.

Baum, C. M., & Edwards, D. (2008). *Activity Card Sort* (2nd ed.). Bethesda, MD: AOTA Press.

Bentzel, K. (2008). Assessing abilities and capacities: Sensation. In M. Radomski & C. Trombly Latham (Eds.), *Occupational therapy for physical dysfunction* (6th ed., pp. 212–233). Philadelphia: Lippincott Williams & Wilkins.

Berg, J. (1997). Playing the outcomes game. *OT Week, 11(22),* 12–15.

Berg, K., Wood-Dauphinee, S., & Williams, J. I. (1995). The Balance Scale: Reliability assessment with elderly residents and patients with an acute stroke. *Scandinavian Journal of Rehabilitative Medicine, 27,* 27–36.

Berger, S., McAteer, J., Schreier, K., & Kaldenberg, J. (2013). Occupational therapy interventions to improve leisure and social participation for older adults with low vision: A systematic review (Suppl. Table 1). *American Journal of Occupational Therapy, 67,* 303–311. http://dx.doi.org/10.5014/ajot.005447

Birk, T., Hickl, S., Wahl, H. W., Miller, D., Kämmerer, A., Holz, F., . . . Völcker, H. E. (2004). Development and pilot evaluation of a psychosocial intervention program for patients with age-related macular degeneration. *Gerontologist, 44,* 836–843. http://dx.doi.org/10.1093/geront/44.6.836

Bowers, A. R., Apfelbaum, D. H., & Peli, E. (2005). Bioptic telescopes meet the needs of drivers with moderate visual acuity loss. *Investigative Ophthalmology and Visual Science, 46,* 66–74. http://dx.doi.org/10.1167/iovs.04-0271

Bowers, A. R., Keeney, K., & Peli, E. (2008). Community-based trial of a peripheral prism visual field expansion device for hemianopia. *Archives of Ophthalmology, 126*(5), 657–664. http://dx.doi.org/10.1001/archopht.126.5.657

Bowers, A. R., Lovie-Kitchin, J. E., & Woods, R. L. (2001). Eye movements and reading with large print and optical magnifiers in macular disease. *Optometry and Vision Science, 78,* 325–334. http://dx.doi.org/10.1097/00006324-200105000-00016

Bowers, A. R., Meek, C., & Stewart, N. (2001). Illumination and reading performance in age-related macular degeneration. *Clinical and Experimental Optometry, 84,* 139–147. http://dx.doi.org/10.1111/j.1444-0938.2001.tb04957.x

Bowers, A., Peli, E., Elgin, J., McGwin, G., Jr., & Owsley, C. (2005). On-road driving with moderate visual field loss. *Optometry and Vision Science, 82,* 657–667. http://dx.doi.org/10.1097/01.opx.0000175558.33268.b5

Boyce, P. B., & Sanford, L. J. (2000). Lighting to enhance visual capabilities. In B. Silverstone, M. A. Lang, B. P. Rosenthal, & E. E. Faye (Eds.), *The Lighthouse handbook on vision impairment and vision rehabilitation* (pp. 617–636). New York: Oxford University Press.

Brody, B. L., Roch-Levecq, A. C., Gamst, A. C., Maclean, K., Kaplan, R. M., & Brown, S. I. (2002). Self-management of age-related macular degeneration and quality of life: A randomized controlled trial. *Archives of Ophthalmology, 120,* 1477–1483.

Brody, B. L., Roch-Levecq, A. C., Thomas, R. G., Kaplan, R. M., & Brown, S. I. (2005). Self-management of age-related macular degeneration at the 6-month follow-up: A randomized controlled trial. *Archives of Ophthalmology, 123,* 46–53. http://dx.doi.org/10.1001/archopht.123.1.46

Brody, B. L., Williams, R. A., Thomas, R. G., Kaplan, R. M., Chu, R. M., & Brown, S. I. (1999). Age-related macular degeneration: A randomized clinical trial of a self-management intervention. *Annals of Behavioral Medicine, 21,* 322–329. http://dx.doi.org/10.1007/BF02895965

Brunnström, G., Sörensen, S., Alsterstad, K., & Sjöstrand, J. (2004). Quality of light and quality of life—The effect of lighting adaptation among people with low vision. *Ophthalmic and Physiological Optics, 24,* 274–280. http://dx.doi.org/10.1111/j.1475-1313.2004.00192.x

Centers for Medicare and Medicaid Services. (2002). *Program memorandum: Intermediaries/carriers* (Transmittal AB-02-078). Retrieved August 25, 2011, from www.cms.gov/Transmittals/downloads/AB02078.pdf

Cheong, A. M., Bowers, A. R., & Lovie-Kitchin, J. E. (2009). Does a line guide improve reading performance with stand magnifiers. *Optometry and Vision Science, 86,* E1078–E1085. http://dx.doi.org/10.1097/OPX.0b013e3181b4c4d9

Cheong, A. M., Lovie-Kitchin, J. E., Bowers, A. R., & Brown, B. (2005). Short-term in-office practice improves reading performance with stand magnifiers for people with AMD. *Optometry and Vision Science, 82,* 114–127. http://dx.doi.org/10.1097/01.OPX.0000153244.93582.FF

Coleman, A. L., Stone, K., Ewing, S. K., Nevitt, M., Cummings, S., Cauley, J. A., . . . Mangione, C. M. (2004). Higher risk of multiple falls among elderly women who lose visual acuity. *Ophthalmology, 111,* 857–862. http://dx.doi.org/10.1016/j.ophtha.2003.09.033

Colenbrander, A. (2002). Visual standards: Aspects and ranges of vision loss. *Proceedings of the 29th International Congress of Ophthamology,* Sydney, Australia. Retrieved from http://www.ski.org/Colenbrander/Images/Vis_Standards_ICO_2002.pdf

Colenbrander, A., & Fletcher, D. C. (1995). Basic concepts and terms for low vision rehabilitation. *American Journal of Occupational Therapy, 49,* 865–869.

Congdon, N., O'Colmain, B., Klaver, C. C., Klein, R., Muñoz, B., Friedman, D. S., . . . Mitchell, P.; Eye Diseases Prevalence Research Group. (2004). Causes and prevalence of visual impairment among adults in the United States. *Archives of Ophthalmology, 122,* 477–485. http://dx.doi.org/10.1001/archopht.122.4.477

Conrod, B. E., & Overbury, O. (1998). The effectiveness of perceptual training and psychosocial counseling in adjustment to the loss of vision. *Journal of Visual Impairment and Blindness, 92,* 464–482.

Crossland, M. D., Culham, L. E., Kabanarou, S. A., & Rubin, G. S. (2005). Preferred retinal locus development in patients with macular disease. *Ophthalmology, 112,* 1579–1585. http://dx.doi.org/10.1016/j.ophtha.2005.03.027

Culham, L. E., Chabra, A., & Rubin, G. S. (2004). Clinical performance of electronic, head-mounted, low-vision devices. *Ophthalmic and Physiological Optics, 24,* 281–290. http://dx.doi.org/10.1111/j.1475-1313.2004.00193.x

Dahlin Ivanoff, S., Sonn, U., & Svensson, E. (2002). A health education program for elderly persons with visual impairments and perceived security in the performance of daily occupations: A randomized study. *American Journal of Occupational Therapy, 56,* 322–330. http://dx.doi.org/10.5014/ajot.56.3.322

de Boer, M. R., Twisk, J., Moll, A. C., Völker-Dieben, H. J. M., de Vet, H. C. W., & van Rens, G. H. M. B. (2006). Outcomes of low-vision services using optometric and multidisciplinary approaches: A non-randomized comparison. *Ophthalmic and Physiological Optics, 26,* 535–544.

Desrosiers, J., Wanet-Defalque, M. C., Témisjian, K., Gresset, J., Dubois, M. F., Renaud, J., . . . Overbury, O. (2009). Participation in daily activities and social roles of older adults with visual impairment. *Disability and Rehabilitation, 31,* 1227–1234. http://dx.doi.org/10.1080/09638280802532456

Dragon Naturally Speaking Speech Recognition Software (Version 12) [Computer software]. Burlington, MA: Nuance Communications.

Duncan, P. W., Weiner, D. K., Chandler, J., & Studenski, S. (1990). Functional reach: A new clinical measure of balance. *Journal of Gerontology, 45,* M192–M197. http://dx.doi.org/10.1093/geronj/45.6.M192

Dunn, W., McClain, L. H., Brown, C., & Youngstrom, M. J. (1998). The ecology of human performance. In M. E. Neistadt & E. B. Crepeau (Eds.), *Willard and Spackman's occupational therapy* (9th ed., pp. 525–535). Philadelphia: Lippincott Williams & Wilkins.

Eklund, K., & Dahlin-Ivanoff, S. (2007). Low vision, ADL and hearing assistive device use among older persons with visual impairments. *Disability and Rehabilitation: Assistive Technology, 2,* 326–334. http://dx.doi.org/10.1080/17483100701714717

Eklund, K., Sjöstrand, J., & Dahlin-Ivanoff, S. (2008). A randomized controlled trial of a health-promotion programme and its effect on ADL dependence and self-reported health problems for the elderly visually impaired. *Scandinavian Journal of Occupational Therapy, 15,* 68–74. http://dx.doi.org/10.1080/11038120701442963

Eklund, K., Sonn, U., & Dahlin-Ivanoff, S. (2004). Long-term evaluation of a health education programme for elderly persons with visual impairment: A randomized study. *Disability and Rehabilitation, 26,* 401–409. http://dx.doi.org/10.1080/09638280410001662950

Elliott, J. L., & Kuyk, T. K. (1994). Self-reported functional and psychosocial outcomes of blind rehabilitation. *Journal of Visual Impairment and Blindness, 88,* 206–212.

Eldred, K. B. (1992). Optimal illumination for reading in patients with age-related maculopathy. *Optometry and Vision Science, 69,* 46–50. http://dx.doi.org/10.1097/00006324-199201000-00007

Engel, R. J., Welsh, R. L., & Lewis, L. J. (2000). Improving the well-being of vision-impaired older adults through orientation and mobility training and rehabilitation. *Evaluation Review, 32,* 67–76.

Eperjesi, F., Fowler, C. W., & Evans, B. J. (2004). The effects of coloured light filter overlays on reading rates in age-related macular degeneration. *Acta Ophthalmologica Scandinavica, 82,* 695–700. http://dx.doi.org/10.1111/j.1600-0420.2004.00371.x

Eperjesi, F., Maiz-Fernandez, C., & Bartlett, H. E. (2007). Reading performance with various lamps in age-related macular degeneration. *Ophthalmic and Physiological Optics, 27,* 93–99.

Figueiro, M. G. (2001). *Lighting the way: A key to independence.* Troy, NY: Lighting Research Center.

Fok, D., Polgar, J. M., Shaw, L., & Jutai, J. W. (2011). Low vision assistive technology device usage and importance in daily occupations. *Work, 39,* 37–48.

Folstein, M. F., Folstein, S. E., & McHugh, P. R. (1975). "Mini-Mental State": A practical method for grading the cognitive state of patients for the clinician. *Journal of Psychiatric Research, 12,* 189–198. http://dx.doi.org/10.1016/0022-3956(75)90026-6

Fosse, P., & Valberg, A. (2004). Lighting needs and lighting comfort during reading with age-related macular degeneration. *Journal of Visual Impairment and Blindness, 98,* 389–409.

Frennesson, C., Jakobsson, P., & Nilsson, U. L. (1995). A computer and video display based system for training eccentric viewing in macular degeneration with an absolute central scotoma. *Documenta Ophthalmologica, 91,* 9–16. http://dx.doi.org/10.1007/BF01204619

Garzia, R. P., Richman, J. E., Nicholson, S. B., & Gaines, C. S. (1990). A new visual–verbal saccade test: The Development Eye Movement test (DEM). *Journal of the American Optometric Association, 61,* 124–135.

Gense, D. J., & Gense, M. (2004). *The importance of orientation and mobility skills for students who are deaf-blind.* Monmouth, OR: DB-LINK. Retrieved April 15, 2012, from http://c324175.r75.cf1.rackcdn.com/products/o&m.pdf

Gilbert, M. P., & Baker, S. S. (2011). Evaluation and intervention for basic and instrumental activities of daily living. In M. Warren & E. A. Barstow (Eds.), *Occupational therapy interventions for adults with low vision* (pp. 227–268). Bethesda, MD: AOTA Press.

Girdler, S. J., Boldy, D. P., Dhaliwal, S. S., Crowley, M., & Packer, T. L. (2010). Vision self management for older adults: A randomized controlled trial. *British Journal of Ophthalmology, 94,* 223–228.

Girdler, S., Packer, T. L., & Boldy, D. (2008). The impact of age-related vision loss: A focus group study. *OTJR: Occupation, Participation and Health, 28,* 110–120. http://dx.doi.org/10.3928/15394492-20080601-05

Golisz, K. (2009). *Occupational therapy practice guidelines for adults with traumatic brain injury.* Bethesda, MD: AOTA Press.

Goodrich, G. L., & Kirby, J. (2001). A comparison of patient reading performance and preference: Optical devices, handheld CCTV (Innoventions Magni-Cam), or stand-mounted CCTV (Optelec Clearview or TSI Genie). *Optometry, 72,* 519–528.

Goodrich, G., Kirby, J., Wagstaff, P., Oros, T., & McDevitt, B. (2004). A comparative study of reading performance with a head-mounted laser display and conventional low vision devices. *Journal of Visual Impairment and Blindness, 98,* 148–159.

Goodrich, G., Kirby, J., Wood, J., & Peters, L. (2006). The Reading Behavior Inventory: An outcome assessment tool. *Journal of Visual Impairment and Blindness, 100,* 164–168.

Hassell, J. B., Lamoureux, E. L., & Keeffe, J. E. (2006). Impact of age related macular degeneration on quality of life. *British Journal of Ophthalmology, 90,* 593–596. http://dx.doi.org/10.1136/bjo.2005.086595

Haymes, S. A., Johnston, A. W., & Heyes, A. D. (2001). The development of the Melbourne Low-Vision ADL Index: A measure of vision disability. *Investigative Ophthalmology and Visual Science, 42,* 1215–1225.

Haymes, S. A., & Lee, J. (2006). Effects of task lighting on visual function in age-related macular degeneration. *Ophthalmic and Physiological Optics, 26,* 169–179. http://dx.doi.org/10.1111/j.1475-1313.2006.00367.x

Hinds, A., Sinclair, A., Park, J., Suttie, A., Paterson, H., & Macdonald, M. (2003). Impact of an interdisciplinary low vision service on the quality of life of low vision patients. *British Journal of Ophthalmology, 87,* 1391–1396. http://dx.doi.org/10.1136/bjo.87.11.1391

Holm, M. B. (2000). Our mandate for the new millennium: Evidence-based practice (Eleanor Clarke Slagle lecture). *American Journal of Occupational Therapy, 54*, 575–585. http://dx.doi .org/10.5014/ajot.54.6.575

Horowitz, A., Brennan, M., Reinhardt, J. P., & Macmillan, T. (2006). The impact of assistive device use on disability and depression among older adults with age-related vision impairments. *Journals of Gerontology, Series B: Psychological Sciences and Social Sciences, 61*, S274–S280.

Horowitz, A., & Reinhardt, J. P. (2000). Mental health issues in vision impairment: Research in depression, disability, and rehabilitation. In B. Silverstone, M. A. Long, B. P. Rosenthal, & E. F. Faye (Eds.), *The Lighthouse handbook of vision impairment and vision rehabilitation* (pp. 1089–1109). New York: Oxford University Press.

Horowitz, A., Teresi, J., & Cassels, L. A. (1991). Development of a vision screening questionnaire for older people. *Journal of Gerontological Social Work, 17*, 37–56. http://dx.doi.org/10.1300/ J083v17n03_04

Humphry, R. C., & Thompson, G. M. (1986). Low vision aids—Evaluation in a general eye department. *Transactions of the Ophthalmological Society of the United Kingdom, 105*, 296–303.

Illuminating Engineering Society of North America. (2007). *Lighting and the visual environment for senior living.* New York: Author.

Itzkovish, M., Elazar, B., & Averbuch, S. (1990). *Loewenstein Occupational Therapy Cognitive Assessment (LOTCA) manual.* Pequannock, NJ: Maddak.

Ivers, R. Q., Cumming, R. G., Mitchell, P., Simpson, J. M., & Peduto, A. J. (2003). Visual risk factors for hip fracture in older people. *Journal of the American Geriatrics Society, 51*, 356–363. http://dx.doi.org/10.1046/j.1532-5415.2003.51109.x

Jaws for Windows: Screen Reading Software (Version 5.0) [Computer software]. St. Petersburg, FL: Freedom Scientific.

Justiss, M. D. (2013). Occupational therapy interventions to promote driving and community mobility for older adults with low vision: A systematic review (Suppl. Table 1). *American Journal of Occupational Therapy, 67*, 296–307. http://dx.doi. org/10.5014/ajot.005660

Jutai, J. W., Strong, G., & Russell-Minda, E. (2009). Effectiveness of assistive technologies for low vision rehabilitation: A systematic review. *Journal of Visual Impairment and Blindness, 103*, 210–222.

Kabanarou, S. A., & Rubin, G. S. (2006). Reading with central scotomas: Is there a binocular gain. *Optometry and Vision Science, 83*, 789–796. http://dx.doi.org/10.1097/01. opx.0000238642.65218.64

Katzman, R., Brown, T., Fuld, P., Peck, A., Schechter, R., & Schimmel, H. (1983). Validation of a short Orientation–Memory–Concentration Test of cognitive impairment. *American Journal of Psychiatry, 140*, 734–739.

Keeffe, J. E., Lam, D., Cheung, A., Dinh, T., & McCarty, C. A. (1998). Impact of vision impairment on functioning. *Australian and New Zealand Journal of Ophthalmology, 26*(Suppl. 1), S16–S18. http://dx.doi.org/10.1111/j.1442-9071.1998. tb01360.x

Kern, T., & Miller, N. (1997). Occupational therapy and collaborative interventions for adults with low vision. In M. Gentile (Ed.), *Functional visual behavior: A therapist's guide to evaluation and treatment options* (pp. 493–535). Bethesda, MD: American Occupational Therapy Association.

Kulp, M. T., & Schmidt, P. P. (1997). Reliability of the NYSOA King–Devick saccadic eye movement test in kindergartners and first graders. *Journal of the American Optometric Association, 68,* 589–594.

Laderman, D. J., Szlyk, J. P., Kelsch, R., & Seiple, W. (2000). A curriculum for training patients with peripheral visual field loss to use bioptic amorphic lenses. *Journal of Rehabilitation Research and Development, 37,* 607–619.

La Grow, S. (2004). The effectiveness of comprehensive low vision services for older persons with visual impairments in New Zealand. *Journal of Visual Impairment and Blindness, 98,* 679–692.

Lamoureux, E. L., Hassell, J. B., & Keeffe, J. E. (2004). The impact of diabetic retinopathy on participation in daily living. *Archives of Ophthalmology, 122,* 84–88. http://dx.doi.org/10.1001/archopht.122.1.84

Lamoureux, E. L., Pallant, J. F., Pesudovs, K., Rees, G., Hassell, J. B., & Keeffe, J. E. (2007). The effectiveness of low-vision rehabilitation on participation in daily living and quality of life. *Investigative Ophthalmology and Visual Science, 48,* 1476–1482. http://dx.doi.org/10.1167/iovs.06-0610

Law, M., Baptiste, S., Carswell, A., McColl, M., Polatajko, H., & Pollock, N. (2004). *COPM: Questions and answers.* Retrieved from https://www.caot.ca/copm/questions.html#15

Law, M., Baptiste, S., Carswell, A., McColl, M., Polatajko, H., & Pollock, N. (2005). *Canadian Occupational Performance Measure manual* (4th ed.). Ottawa, Ontario: CAOT Publications.

Law, M., Baptiste, S., McColl, M. A., Opzoomer, A., Polatajko, H., & Pollock, N. (1990). The Canadian Occupational Performance Measure: An outcome measure for occupational therapy. *Canadian Journal of Occupational Therapy, 57,* 82–87.

Law, M., & Baum, C. (1998). Evidence-based occupational therapy. *Canadian Journal of Occupational Therapy, 65,* 131–135.

Lee, H. K. M., & Scudds, R. J. (2003). Comparison of balance in older people with and without visual impairment. *Age and Ageing, 32,* 643–649. http://dx.doi.org/10.1093/ageing/afg110

Lieberman, D., & Scheer, J. (2002). AOTA's evidence-based literature review project: An overview. *American Journal of Occupational Therapy, 56,* 344–349. http://dx.doi.org/10.5014/ajot.56.3.344

Lighthouse International. (1996). *Functional Vision Screening Questionnaire.* Retrieved November 3, 2011, from www.aoa.org/documents/POA-Lighthouse-International-Functional-Vision-Screening-Questionnaire.pdf

Liu, C.-J., Brost, M. A., Horton, V. E., Kenyon, S. B., & Mears, K. E. (2013). Occupational therapy interventions to improve performance of daily activities at home for older adults with low vision: A systematic review (Suppl. Table 1). *American Journal of Occupational Therapy, 67,* 279–287. http://dx.doi.org/10.5014/ajot.005512

List of Impairments, 20 C.F.R. Ch. III, Pt. 404, Subpt. P, App. 1. (2006).

Lord, S. R. (2006). Visual risk factors for falls in older people. *Age and Ageing, 35*(Suppl. 2), ii42–ii45. http://dx.doi.org/10.1093/ageing/afl085

Lord, S. R., & Dayhew, J. (2001). Visual risk factors for falls in older people. *Journal of the American Geriatrics Society, 49,* 508–515. http://dx.doi.org/10.1046/j.1532-5415.2001.49107.x

Mahoney, F. I., & Barthel, D. W. (1965). Functional evaluation: The Barthel Index. *Maryland State Medical Journal, 14,* 61–65.

Mangione, C. M., Gutierrez, P. R., Lowe, G., Orav, E. J., & Seddon, J. M. (1999). Influence of age-related maculopathy on visual functioning and health-related quality of life. *American Journal of Ophthalmology, 128*(1), 45–53.

Mangione, C. M., Lee, P. P., Gutierrez, P. R., Spritzer, K., Berry, S., & Hays, R. D.; National Eye Institute Visual Function Questionnaire Field Test Investigators. (2001). Development of the 25-item National Eye Institute Visual Function Questionnaire. *Archives of Ophthalmology, 119,* 1050–1058.

Mann, W. C., Goodall, S., Justiss, M. D., & Tomita, M. (2002). Dissatisfaction and nonuse of assistive devices among frail elders. *Assistive Technology, 14,* 130–139. http://dx.doi.org/10.1080/10400435.2002.10132062

Mansfield, J. S., Legge, G. E., Luebker, A., & Cunningham, K. (1994). *MNRead Acuity Charts: Continuous-text reading-acuity charts for normal and low vision.* Long Island City, NY: Lighthouse Low Vision Products.

Maples, W. C., Atchley, J., & Ficklin, T. (1992). Northeastern State University College of Optometry's oculomotor norms. *Journal of Behavioral Optometry, 3,* 143–150.

Margrain, T. H. (2000). Helping blind and partially sighted people to read: The effectiveness of low vision aids. *British Journal of Ophthalmology, 84,* 919–921. http://dx.doi.org/10.1136/bjo.84.8.919

Markowitz, S. N., Kent, C. K., Schuchard, R. A., & Fletcher, D. C. (2008). Ability to read medication labels improved by participation in a low vision rehabilitation program. *Journal of Visual Impairment and Blindness, 102,* 774–777.

McCabe, P., Nason, F., Demers Turco, P., Friedman, D., & Seddon, J. M. (2000). Evaluating the effectiveness of a vision rehabilitation intervention using an objective and subjective measure of functional performance. *Ophthalmic Epidemiology, 7,* 259–270. http://dx.doi.org/10.1076/opep.7.4.259.4173

McColl, M. A., Carswell, A., Law, M., Pollock, N., Baptiste, S., & Polatajko, H. (2006). *Research on the Canadian Occupational Performance Measure: An annotated resource.* Ottawa, Ontario: CAOT Publications.

McIlwaine, G. G., Bell, J. A., & Dutton, G. N. (1991). Low vision aids—Is our service cost effective? *Eye, 5,* 607–611. http://dx.doi.org/10.1038/eye.1991.105

Minkel, J. L. (1996). Assistive technology and outcome measurement: Where do we begin? *Technology and Disability, 5,* 285–288. http://dx.doi.org/10.1016/S1055-4181(96)00175-6

Moyers, P., & Dale, L. (2007). *The guide to occupational therapy practice* (2nd ed.). Bethesda, MD: AOTA Press.

Nasreddine, Z. (2011). *Montreal Cognitive Assessment.* Retrieved November 4, 2011, from www.mocatest.org

National Eye Institute. (2009a). *Facts about age-related macular degeneration.* Retrieved September 2, 2011, from www.nei.nih.gov/health/maculardegen/armd_facts.asp

National Eye Institute. (2009b). *Facts about cataract.* Retrieved September 2, 2011, from www.nei.nih.gov/health/cataract/cataract_facts.asp

National Eye Institute. (2009c). *Facts about diabetic retinopathy.* Retrieved September 2, 2011, from www.nei.nih.gov/health/diabetic/retinopathy.asp

National Eye Institute. (2011). *Glaucoma.* Retrieved October 22, 2012, from http://report.nih.gov/NIHfactsheets/ViewFactSheet.aspx?csid=92&key=G#G

National Eye Institute. (n.d.). *What you should know about low vision*. Retrieved October 28, 2012, from www.nei.nih.gov/health/lowvision/Low VisPatBro2.pdf

Nguyen, N. X., Weismann, M., & Trauzettel-Klosinski, S. (2009). Improvement of reading speed after providing of low vision aids in patients with age-related macular degeneration. *Acta Ophthalmologica, 87*, 849–853. http://dx.doi.org/10.1111/j.1755-3768.2008.01423.x

Nilsson, U. (1990). Visual rehabilitation with and without educational training in the use of optical aids and residual vision: A prospective study of patients with advanced age-related macular degeneration. *Clinical Vision Sciences, 6*, 3–10.

Noell-Waggoner, E. (2004). Lighting solutions for contemporary problems of older adults. *Psychosocial Nursing and Mental Health Services, 42*, 14–20.

Owsley, C., McGwin, G., Jr., Lee, P. P., Wasserman, N., & Searcey, K. (2009). Characteristics of low-vision rehabilitation services in the United States. *Archives of Ophthalmology, 127*, 681–689. http://dx.doi.org/10.1001/archophthalmol.2009.55

Owsley, C., McGwin, G., Jr., Phillips, J. M., McNeal, S. F., & Stalvey, B. T. (2004). Impact of an educational program on the safety of high-risk, visually impaired, older drivers. *American Journal of Preventive Medicine, 26*, 222–229. http://dx.doi.org/10.1016/j.amepre.2003.12.005

Packer, T. L., Girdler, S., Boldy, D. P., Dhaliwal, S. S., & Crowley, M. (2009). Vision self-management for older adults: A pilot study. *Disability and Rehabilitation, 31*, 1353–1361. http://dx.doi.org/10.1080/09638280802572999

Pankow, L., Luchins, D., Studebaker, J., & Chettleburgh, D. (2004). Evaluation of a vision rehabilitation program for older adults with visual impairment. *Topics in Geriatric Rehabilitation, 20*, 223–235.

Patel, P. J., Chen, F. K., Da Cruz, L., Rubin, G. S., & Tufail, A. (2011). Test–retest variability of reading performance metrics using MNRead in patients with age-related macular degeneration. *Investigative Ophthalmology and Visual Science, 52*, 3854–3859. http://dx.doi.org/10.1167/iovs.10-6601

Perlmutter, M. (n.d.). *Home Environment Lighting Assessment* (3rd ed.). Unpublished instrument.

Perlmutter, M. S., Bhorade, A., Gordon, M., Hollingsworth, H. H., & Baum, M. C. (2010). Cognitive, visual, auditory, and emotional factors that affect participation in older adults. *American Journal of Occupational Therapy, 64*, 570–579. http://dx.doi.org/10.5014/ajot.2010.09089

Peterson, R. C., Wolffsohn, J. S., Rubinstein, M., & Lowe, J. (2003). Benefits of electronic vision enhancement systems (EVES) for the visually impaired. *American Journal of Ophthalmology, 136*, 1129–1135. http://dx.doi.org/10.1016/S0002-9394(03)00567-1

Phillips, B., & Zhao, H. (1993). Predictors of assistive technology abandonment. *Assistive Technology, 5*, 36–45. http://dx.doi.org/10.1080/10400435.1993.10132205

Pizzimenti, J. J., & Roberts, E. (2005, July). The low vision rehabilitation service: Part two. Putting the program into practice. *Internet Journal of Allied Health Science and Practice, 3*(3). Retrieved November 16, 2011, from http://ijahsp.nova.edu/articles/vol3num3/Pizzimenti_Roberts.htm

Podsiadlo, D., & Richardson, S. (1991). The Timed "Up & Go": A test of basic functional mobility for frail elderly persons. *Journal of the American Geriatrics Society, 39*, 142–148.

Quintana, L. (2008). Assessing abilities and capacities: Vision, visual perception, and praxis. In M. Radomski & C. Trombly Latham (Eds.), *Occupational therapy for physical dysfunction* (6th ed., pp. 234–259). Philadelphia: Lippincott Williams & Wilkins.

Radloff, L. S. (1977). The CES–D scale: A self-report depression scale for research in the general population. *Applied Psychological Measurement, 1,* 385–401. http://dx.doi.org/10.1177/014662167700100306

Ramrattan, R. S., Wolfs, R. C., Panda-Jonas, S., Jonas, J. B., Bakker, D., Pols, H. A., . . . de Jong, P. T. (2001). Prevalence and causes of visual field loss in the elderly and associations with impairment in daily functioning: The Rotterdam Study. *Archives of Ophthalmology, 119,* 1788–1794.

Reeves, B. C., Harper, R. A., & Russell, W. B. (2004). Enhanced low vision rehabilitation for people with age related macular degeneration: A randomised controlled trial. *British Journal of Ophthalmology, 88,* 1443–1449. http://dx.doi.org/10.1136/bjo.2003.037457

Rein, D. B., Wittenborn, J. S., Zhang, X., Honeycutt, A. A., Lesesne, S. B., & Saaddine, J.; Vision Health Cost-Effectiveness Study Group. (2009). Forecasting age-related macular degeneration through the year 2050: The potential impact of new treatments. *Archives of Ophthalmology, 127,* 533–540. http://dx.doi.org/10.1001/archophthalmol.2009.58

Riemer-Reiss, M. L., & Wacker, R. R. (2000). Factors associated with assistive technology discontinuance among individuals with disabilities. *Journal of Rehabilitation, 66,* 44–50.

Rovner, B. W., & Casten, R. J. (2008). Preventing late-life depression in age-related macular degeneration. *American Journal of Geriatric Psychiatry, 16,* 454–459. http://dx.doi.org/10.1097/JGP.0b013e31816b7342

Rovner, B. W., Casten, R. J., & Tasman, W. S. (2002). Effect of depression on vision function in age-related macular degeneration. *Archives of Ophthalmology, 120,* 1041–1044. http://dx.doi.org/10.1001/archopht.120.8.1041

Rubin, G. S., Roche, K. B., Prasada-Rao, P., & Fried, L. P. (1994). Visual impairment and disability in older adults. *Optometry and Vision Science, 71,* 750–760. http://dx.doi.org/10.1097/00006324-199412000-00005

Russell-Minda, E., Jutai, J. W., Strong, G., Campbell, K. A., Gold, D., Pretty, L., & Wilmot, L. (2007). The legibility of typefaces for readers with low vision: A research review. *Journal of Visual Impairment and Blindness, 101,* 402–415.

Rustad, R. A., DeGroot, T. L., Jungkunz, M. L., Freeberg, K. S., Borowick, L. G., & Wanttie, A. M. (1993). *The Cognitive Assessment of Minnesota.* Tucson, AZ: Therapy Skill Builders.

Saaddine, J. B., Honeycutt, A. A., Narayan, K. M., Zhang, X., Klein, R., & Boyle, J. P. (2008). Projection of diabetic retinopathy and other major eye diseases among people with diabetes mellitus: United States, 2005–2050. *Archives of Ophthalmology, 126,* 1740–1747. http://dx.doi.org/10.1001/archopht.126.12.1740

Sabari, J. (2008). *Occupational therapy practice guidelines for adults with stroke.* Bethesda, MD: AOTA Press.

Sackett, D. L., Rosenberg, W. M., Muir Gray, J. A., Haynes, R. B., & Richardson, W. S. (1996). Evidence–based medicine: What it is and what it isn't. *British Medical Journal, 312,* 71–72. http://dx.doi.org/10.1136/bmj.312.7023.71

Sanford, L. (1997). Guidelines for designing lighting for the elderly. *Lighting Management and Maintenance, 25*(6), 14–15, 28–29.

Scanlan, J. M., & Cuddeford, J. E. (2004). Low vision rehabilitation: A comparison of traditional and extended teaching programs. *Journal of Visual Impairment and Blindness, 98,* 601–611.

Scheiman, M. (2002). *Understanding and managing vision deficits: A guide for occupational therapists* (2nd ed.). Thorofare, NJ: Slack.

Scheiman, M., Scheiman, M., & Whittaker, S. (2007). *Low vision rehabilitation: A practical guide for occupational therapists.* Thorofare, NJ: Slack.

Schuchard, R. A. (2005). Preferred retinal loci and macular scotoma characteristics in patients with age-related macular degeneration. *Canadian Journal of Ophthalmology, 40,* 303–312.

Scott, I. U., Schein, O. D., Feuer, W. J., Folstein, M. F., & Bandeen-Roche, K. (2001). Emotional distress in patients with retinal disease. *American Journal of Ophthalmology, 131*(5), 584–589.

Shuttleworth, G. N., Dunlop, A., Collins, J. K., & James, C. R. H. (1995). How effective is an integrated approach to low vision rehabilitation? Two year follow up results from south Devon. *British Journal of Ophthalmology, 79,* 719–723. http://dx.doi.org/10.1136/bjo.79.8.719

Skelton, D. A. (2001). Effects of physical activity on postural stability. *Age and Ageing, 30*(Suppl. 4), 33–39. http://dx.doi.org/10.1093/ageing/30.suppl_4.33

Slakter, J. S., & Stur, M. (2005). Quality of life in patients with age-related macular degeneration: Impact of the condition and benefits of treatment. *Survey of Ophthalmology, 50,* 263–273. http://dx.doi.org/10.1016/j.survophthal.2005.02.007

Smallfield, S., Schaefer, K., & Myers, A. (2013). Occupational therapy interventions to improve the reading ability of older adults with low vision: A systematic review (Suppl. Table 1). *American Journal of Occupational Therapy, 67,* 288–295. http://dx.doi.org/10.5014/ajot.004929

Smith, H. J., Dickinson, C. M., Cacho, I., Reeves, B. C., & Harper, R. A. (2005). A randomized controlled trial to determine the effectiveness of prism spectacles for patients with age-related macular degeneration. *Archives of Ophthalmology, 123,* 1042–1050. http://dx.doi.org/10.1001/archopht.123.8.1042

Sokol-McKay, D., Buskirk, K., & Whittaker, P. (2003). Adaptive low-vision and blindness techniques for blood glucose monitoring. *Diabetes Educator, 29,* 614–618, 620, 622. http://dx.do.org/10.1177/014572170302900408

Sokol-McKay, D. A., & Michels, D. (2005, May 23). Facing the challenge of macular degeneration: Therapeutic interventions for low vision. *OT Practice, 10,* 10–15.

Spitzer, R. L., Kroenke, K., & Williams, J. B. (1999). Validation and utility of a self-report version of PRIME–MD: The PHQ primary care study. Primary care evaluation of mental disorders. Patient Health Questionnaire. *JAMA, 282,* 1737–1744. http://dx.doi.org/10.1001/jama.282.18.1737

Stalvey, B. T., & Owsley, C. (2003). The development and efficacy of a theory-based educational curriculum to promote self-regulation among high-risk older drivers. *Health Promotion Practice, 4,* 109–119.

Stav, W. B., Hunt, L. A., & Arbesman, M. (2006). *Occupational therapy practice guidelines for driving and community mobility for older adults.* Bethesda, MD: AOTA Press.

Stelmack, J. A., Moran, D., Dean, D., & Massof, R. W. (2007). Short- and long-term effects of an intensive inpatient vision rehabilitation program. *Archives of Physical Medicine and Rehabilitation, 88,* 691–695. http://dx.doi.org/10.1016/j.apmr.2007.03.025

Stelmack, J., Reda, D., Ahlers, S., Bainbridge, L., & McCray, J. (1991). Reading performance of geriatric patients post exudative maculopathy. *Journal of the American Optometric Association, 62,* 53–57.

Stelmack, J. A., Tang, X. C., Reda, D. J., Rinne, S., Mancil, R. M., & Massof, R. W.; LOVIT Study Group. (2008). Outcomes of the Veterans Affairs Low Vision Intervention Trial (LOVIT). *Archives of Ophthalmology, 126,* 608–617. http://dx.doi.org/10.1001/archopht.126.5.608

Stevens-Ratchford, R., & Krause, A. (2004). Visually impaired older adults and home-based leisure activities: The effects of person–environment congruence. *Journal of Visual Impairment and Blindness, 98,* 14–27.

Studebaker, J., & Pankow, L. (2004). History and evolution of vision rehabilitation: Parallels with rehabilitation medicine, geriatric medicine, and psychiatry. *Topics in Geriatric Rehabilitation, 20,* 142–153.

Stuen, C., & Faye, E. (2003). Vision loss: Normal and not normal changes among older adults. *Generations, 27,* 8–14.

Subramanian, A., & Pardhan, S. (2006). The repeatability of MNRead acuity charts and variability at different test distances. *Optometry and Vision Science, 83,* 572–576. http://dx.doi.org/10.1097/01.opx.0000232225.00311.53

Szlyk, J. P., Seiple, W., Laderman, D. J., Kelsch, R., Ho, K., & McMahon, T. (1998). Use of bioptic amorphic lenses to expand the visual field in patients with peripheral loss. *Optometry and Vision Science, 75,* 518–524. http://dx.doi.org/10.1097/00006324-199807000-00021

Szlyk, J. P., Seiple, W., Laderman, D. J., Kelsch, R., Stelmack, J., & McMahon, T. (2000). Measuring the effectiveness of bioptic telescopes for persons with central vision loss. *Journal of Rehabilitation Research and Development, 37,* 101–108.

Szlyk, J. P., Seiple, W., Stelmack, J., & McMahon, T. (2005). Use of prisms for navigation and driving in hemianopic patients. *Ophthalmic and Physiological Optics, 25,* 128–135. http://dx.doi.org/10.1111/j.1475-1313.2004.00265.x

Taylor, H. R. (2002). Eye care for the community. *Clinical and Experimental Ophthalmology, 30,* 151–154. http://dx.doi.org/10.1046/j.1442-9071.2002.00525.x

Teitelman, J., & Copolillo, A. (2005). Psychosocial issues in older adults' adjustment to vision loss: Findings from qualitative interviews and focus groups. *American Journal of Occupational Therapy, 59,* 409–417.

Tinetti, M. E. (1986). Performance-oriented assessment of mobility problems in elderly patients. *Journal of the American Geriatrics Society, 34,* 119–126.

Trombly, C. A. (1995). Occupation: Purposefulness and meaningfulness as therapeutic mechanisms. *American Journal of Occupational Therapy, 49,* 960–972.

Uniform Data System for Medical Rehabilitation. (1997). *Guide for the Uniform Data Set for Medical Rehabilitation (including the FIM^{TM} instrument), Version 5.1.* Buffalo: State University of New York at Buffalo.

U.S. Preventive Services Task Force. (2008). *Grade definitions.* Retrieved December 16, 2011, from www.uspreventiveservicestaskforce.org/uspstf/grades.htm

Vukicevic, M., & Fitzmaurice, K. (2005). Rehabilitation strategies used to ameliorate the impact of centre field loss. *Visual Impairment Research, 7,* 79–84. http://dx.doi.org/10.1080/13388235050037762

Vukicevic, M., & Fitzmaurice, K. (2009). Eccentric viewing training in the home environment: Can it improve the performance of activities of daily living? *Journal of Visual Impairment and Blindness, 103,* 277–290.

Waern, M., Rubenowitz, E., Runeson, B., Skoog, I., Wilhelmson, K., & Allebeck, P. (2002). Burden of illness and suicide in elderly people: Case-control study. *British Medical Journal, 324,* 1355–1358. http://dx.doi.org/10.1136/bmj.324.7350.1355

Wang, J. J., Mitchell, P., Simpson, J. M., Cumming, R. G., & Smith, W. (2001). Visual impairment, age-related cataract, and mortality. *Archives of Ophthalmology, 119,* 1186–1190.

Warren, M. (1993a). A hierarchical model for evaluation and treatment of visual perceptual dysfunction in adult acquired brain injury, Part 1. *American Journal of Occupational Therapy, 47,* 42–54. http://dx.doi.org/10.5014/ajot.47.1.42

Warren, M. (1993b). A hierarchical model for evaluation and treatment of visual perceptual dysfunction in adult acquired brain injury, Part 2. *American Journal of Occupational Therapy, 47,* 55–66. http://dx.doi.org/10.5014/ajot.47.1.55

Warren, M. (1998). *Brain Injury Visual Assessment Battery for Adults.* Lenexa, KS: visABILITIES Rehab Services.

Warren, M. (2006). Evaluation and treatment of visual deficits following brain injury. In H. Pendleton & W. Schultz-Krohn (Eds.), *Pedretti's occupational therapy: Practice skills for physical dysfunction* (6th ed., pp. 532–572). St. Louis, MO: Mosby/Elsevier.

Warren, M., & Lampert, J. (1994). Considerations in addressing the daily living needs in older persons with low vision. *Low Vision and Visual Rehabilitation, 7,* 187–195.

Watson, G., Baldasare, J., & Whittaker, S. (1990). Validity and clinical uses of the Pepper Visual Skills for Reading Test. *Journal of Visual Impairment and Blindness, 84,* 119–123.

Watson, G. R., Ramsey, V., De l'Aune, W., & Elk, A. (2004). Ergonomic enhancement for older readers with low vision. *Journal of Visual Impairment and Blindness, 98,* 228–240.

Watson, G. R., Whittaker, S., & Steciw, M. (1995). *The Pepper Visual Skills for Reading Test* (2nd ed.). Lilburn, GA: Bear Consultants.

Watson, G. R., Wright, V., & Long, S. L. (1996). *Morgan Low Vision Reading Comprehension Assessment (LUV Reading Series).* Lilburn, GA: Bear Consultants.

Watson, G. R., Wright, V., Long, S., & De l'Aune, W. (1996). A low vision reading comprehension test. *Journal of Vision Impairment and Blindness, 90,* 486–494.

Watson, G. R., Wright, V., Wyse, E., & De l'Aune, W. (2004). A writing assessment for persons with age-related vision loss. *Journal of Visual Impairment and Blindness, 3,* 160–167.

Weisser-Pike, O., & Kaldenberg, J. (2010). Occupational therapy approaches to facilitate productive aging for individuals with low vision. *OT Practice, 15*(3), CE1–CE8.

West, S. K., Rubin, G. S., Broman, A. T., Muñoz, B., Bandeen-Roche, K., & Turano, K. (2002). How does visual impairment affect performance on tasks of everyday life? The SEE Project. *Archives of Ophthalmology, 120,* 774–780. http://dx.doi.org/10.1001/archopht.120.6.774

Whittle, H., & Goldenberg, D. (1996). Functional health status and instrumental activities of daily living performance in noninstitutionalized elderly people. *Journal of Advanced Nursing, 23,* 220–227.

Williams, R. A., Brody, B. L., Thomas, R. G., Kaplan, R. M., & Brown, S. I. (1998). The psychosocial impact of macular degeneration. *Archives of Ophthalmology, 116*(4), 514–520.

Wolffsohn, J. S., & Cochrane, A. L. (2000). Design of the Low Vision Quality-of-Life Questionnaire (LVQOL) and measuring the outcome of low-vision rehabilitation. *American Journal of Ophthalmology, 130,* 793–802. http://dx.doi.org/10.1016/S0002-9394(00)00610-3

Wolffsohn, J. S., Dinardo, C., & Vingrys, A. J. (2002). Benefit of coloured lenses for age-related macular degeneration. *Ophthalmic and Physiological Optics, 22,* 300–311. http://dx.doi.org/10.1046/j.1475-1313.2002.00036.x

Wolter, M., & Preda, S. (2006). Visual deficits following stroke: Maximizing participation in rehabilitation. *Topics in Stroke Rehabilitation, 13,* 12–21. http://dx.doi.org/10.1310/3JRY-B168-5N49-XQWA

Womack, J. L. (2012, February 20). Continuing life on the move: Aging and community mobility. *OT Practice, 17*(3), CE1–CE8.

World Health Organization. (1999). *International classification of diseases, 9th revision, clinical modification [ICD–9–CM].* Geneva: Author.

World Health Organization. (2001). *International classification of functioning, disability and health.* Geneva: Author.

Yesavage, J. A., Brink, T. L., Rose, T. L., Lum, O., Huang, V., Adey, M., & Leirer, V. O. (1982–1983). Development and validation of a geriatric depression screening scale: A preliminary report. *Journal of Psychiatric Research, 17,* 37–49. http://dx.doi.org/10.1016/0022-3956(82)90033-4

Zoltan, B. (2007). *Vision, perception, and cognition: A manual for the evaluation and treatment of the adult with acquired brain injury* (4th ed.). Thorofare, NJ: Slack.

ZoomText Magnifier/Reader (version 10) [Computer software]. Manchester Center, VT: Ai Squared.

Subject Index

Note: Page numbers in italics indicate figures, boxes, and tables.

rehabilitation
    case study, *11*
    diagnostic codes, 10–11, *10*
    education throughout, 27–28
    evidence tables, *76–77, 82–83*
    team members, *39*
rehabilitation counselors, *40*
research, implications for, 48–49
review, intervention, 44–45

safety, 24
scotoma, 6, 28–30, *29*
    see also age-related eye diseases
screening for functional vision, 9
self-management strategies, 37–39
Self-Report Assessment of Functional Visual
    Performance Profile, 15–16
    see also assessments
sensory substitution strategies, 32–33
services, for organizations and populations, 46–47
social contextual factors, 20–21
social environment, 22
    see also environmental factors
social participation, evidence tables, *87–94*
stand magnifiers, *30*
    see also low vision devices (LVDs)
strong evidence, 62
    see also evidence

systematic reviews, *61*, 63
    see also evidence-based practice (EBP)

teachers for children with visual impairment, *40*
telescopes, *30*
    see also low vision devices (LVDs)
temporal context, 20–21
    see also contextual factors
top-down evaluation, 15
    see also evaluation
typoscopes, 35

virtual environment, 22
    see also environmental factors
vision rehabilitation therapists, *40*
visual efficiency, 19
visual function, 19
visual perception, 19
Visual Skills for Reading Test (VSRT), 18, 45
    see also assessments
visual skills training, 28–30, *29*

writing guides, 35
writing skills, 18–19
    see also psychosocial issues associated with
        visual loss

ZoomText Screen Magnifier/ Reader, 22

Citation Index

Note: Page numbers in italics indicate figures, boxes, and tables.

National Eye Institute [NEI] (2009a), 6, 7
National Eye Institute [NEI] (2009b), 7
National Eye Institute [NEI] (2009c), 8
National Eye Institute [NEI] (2011), 5
NEI (n.d.), 5, 7
Nguyen, Weismann, & Trauzettel- Klosinski (2009), 31, 52, *74*
Nilsson (1990), *70*
Noell-Waggoner (2004), 52

Owsley, McGwin, Lee, Wasserman, & Searcey (2009), 5, 6
Owsley, McGwin, Phillips, McNeal, & Stalvey (2004), 37, *83*

Packer et al. (2009), *68*
Pankow, Luchins, Studebaker, & Chettleburgh (2004), 40, 42, 43, 48, 52, *70, 92*
Patel, Chen, Da Cruz, Rubin, & Tufail (2011), 18
Perlmutter (n.d.), *12*, 21
Perlmutter, Bhorade, Gordon, Hollingsworth, & Baum (2010), 6
Perlmutter et al. (2010), 49
Peterson, Wolffsohn, Rubinstein, & Lowe (2003), 31, 32, 52, *75*
Phillips & Zhao (1993), 31
Pizzimenti & Roberts (2005), 16
Podsiadlo & Richardson (1991), *12*

Quintana (2008), *13*, 19, 28

Radloff (1977), *12*, 17
Ramrattan et al. (2001), 9
Reeves, Harper, & Russell (2004), 43, 44, 48, *71, 92*
Rein et al. (2009), 5
Riemer-Reiss & Wacker (2000), 31
Rovner, Casten & Tasman (2002), 16
Rovner & Casten (2008), 28, 38, 39, 51, *93*
Rubin, Roche, Prasada-Rao, & Fried (1994), 9
Russell-Minda et al. (2007), 35, *80*
Rustad et al. (1993), *12*, 19

Saaddine et al. (2008), 5
Sabari (2008), 6, 8
Sackett, Rosenberg, Muir Gray, Haynes, and Richardson (1996), 59
Sanford (1997), 52
Scanlan & Cuddeford (2004), 43, 44, 48, *71, 77, 93*
Scheiman (2002), *13*
Scheiman, Scheiman, and Whittaker (2007), *40*
Schuchard (2005), 28
Scott, Schein, Feuer, Folstein, & Bandeen-Roche (2001), 16
Shuttleworth, Dunlop, Collins, & James (1995), 44, *94*
Skelton (2001), 36
Slakter & Stur (2005), 16
Smallfield, Schaefer, & Myers (2013), 63
Smith et al. (2005), *72*
Sokol-McKay, Buskirk, & Whittaker (2003), 32
Sokol-McKay and Michels (2005), *40*
Spitzer, Kroenke, & Williams (1999), 17
Stalvey & Owsley (2003), 37, *84*
Stav, Hunt, & Arbesman (2006), 36
Stelmack, Reda, Ahlers, Bainbridge, & McCray (1991), 31, 32, 52
Stelmack et al. (2007), *72*
Stelmack et al. (2008), 43, 44, 48, *72, 78*
Stevens-Ratchford & Krause (2004), 51
Studebaker and Pankow (2004), *40*
Stuen & Faye (2003), 5, 6
Subramanian & Pardhan (2006), 18
Szlyk et al. (1998), 37, *85*
Szlyk et al. (2000), 37, *85*
Szlyk et al. (2005), 37, *86*

Taylor (2002), 9
Teitelman & Copolillo (2005), 16
Tinetti (1986), *12*
Trombly (1995), 3

U.S. Preventive Services Task Force (2008), 27

Vukicevic & Fitzmaurice (2005), 29, *81*

Summary

Although more research is necessary, the results of this evidence-based literature review support the role of occupational therapy with older adults with low vision and provide evidence for the effectiveness of specific occupational therapy interventions. Strong evidence has validated multidisciplinary low vision programs that include occupational therapy, multicomponent education and training for ADLs and IADLs, and training in problem-solving strategies. There is moderately strong evidence substantiating the benefits of electronic magnification and moderate evidence regarding the influence of illumination levels on reading performance and social participation. Finally, there is limited evidence for eccentric viewing training and optical magnification.

The goal of occupational therapy assessment and intervention for older adults with low vision is to maximize the ability to engage in daily occupations in a manner that is client centered, occupation based, and grounded in evidence. Through the provision of education, development of new skills, utilization of adaptive or compensatory strategies, and advocacy for needed services or modifications, older adults with vision loss may be able to maintain their participation in daily activities. Occupational therapy services are a vital component of maintaining the health, well-being, and quality of life of older adults with vision loss.